Handbook of
Drugs in Intensive Care
An A–Z Guide
Fifth Edition

Henry G W Paw
BPharm MRPharmS MBBS FRCA FFICM
Consultant in Intensive Care Medicine and Anaesthesia
York Hospital
York
UK

Rob Shulman
BSc(Pharm) MRPharmS DipClinPharm DHC(Pharm)
Lead Pharmacist in Critical Care
Honorary Associate Professor in Clinical Pharmacy Practice
UCL School of Pharmacy
Honorary Lecturer, Department of Medicine, UCL
University College London Hospitals
London
UK

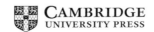
CAMBRIDGE
UNIVERSITY PRESS

CAMBRIDGE
UNIVERSITY PRESS

University Printing House, Cambridge CB2 8BS, United Kingdom

Published in the United States of America by Cambridge University Press, New York

Cambridge University Press is part of the University of Cambridge.

It furthers the University's mission by disseminating knowledge in the pursuit of education, learning and research at the highest international levels of excellence.

www.cambridge.org
Information on this title: www.cambridge.org/9781107484030

First published 2000
Second Edition 2002
Third Edition 2006
Fourth Edition 2009
Fifth Edition 2013
Reprinted with corrections 2014

Printed in the United Kingdom by CPI Group Ltd, Croydon CR0 4YY

A catalogue record for this publication is available from the British Library

Library of Congress Cataloguing in Publication data

ISBN 978-1-107-48403-0 paperback

CONTENTS

APPENDICES   321

DRUG INDEX   339

Inside back cover: IV compatibility chart

INTRODUCTION

Since the publication of the fourth edition in 2010, there have been several new drugs introduced to the critical care setting. This book has now been extensively updated. The main purpose of this book is to provide a practical guide that explains how to use drugs safely and effectively in a critical care setting. Doctors, nurses, pharmacists and other healthcare professionals caring for the critically ill patient will find it useful. It is not intended to list every conceivable complication and problem that can occur with a drug but to concentrate on those the clinician is likely to encounter. The book should be seen as complementary to, rather than replacing, the standard textbooks.

The book is composed of two main sections. The A–Z guide is the major part and is arranged alphabetically by the non-proprietary name of the drug. This format has made it easier for the user to find a particular drug when in a hurry. The discussion on an individual drug is restricted to its use in the critically ill adult patient. The second part is comprised of short notes on relevant intensive care topics. Inside the back cover is a colour fold-out chart showing drug compatibility for intravenous administration.

I am very fortunate to have on board a senior ICU pharmacist for this edition. While every effort has been made to check drug dosages based on a 70 kg adult and information about every drug, it is still possible that errors may have crept in. I would therefore ask readers to check the information if it seems incorrect. In addition, I would be pleased to hear from any readers with suggestions about how this book can be improved. Comments should be sent via e-mail to: henry.paw@york.nhs.uk.

HGWP
York 2013

HOW TO USE THIS BOOK

European law (directive 92/27/EEC) requires the use of the Recommended International Non-proprietary Name (rINN) in place of the British Approved Name (BAN). For a small number of drugs these names are different. The Department of Health requires the use of BAN to cease and be replaced by rINN with the exceptions of adrenaline and noradrenaline. For these two drugs both their BAN and rINN will continue to be used.

The format of this book was chosen to make it more 'user friendly' – allowing the information to be readily available to the reader in times of need. For each drug there is a brief introduction, followed by the following categories:

Uses
This is the indication for the drug's use in the critically ill. There will be some unlicensed use included and this will be indicated in brackets.

Contraindications
This includes conditions or circumstances in which the drug should not be used – the contraindications. For every drug, this includes known hypersensitivity to the particular drug or its constituents.

Administration
This includes the route and dosage for a 70 kg adult. For obese patients, estimated ideal body weight should be used in the calculation of the dosage (Appendix D). It also advises on dilutions and situations where dosage may have to be modified. To make up a dilution, the instruction 'made up to 50 ml with 0.9% sodium chloride' means that the final volume is 50 ml. In contrast, the instruction 'to dilute with 50 ml 0.9% sodium chloride' could result in a total volume >50 ml. It is recommended that no drug should be stored for >24 h after reconstitution or dilution.

How not to use …
Describes administration techniques or solutions for dilution which are not recommended.

Adverse effects
These are effects other than those desired.

Cautions
Warns of situations when the use of the drug is not contraindicated but needs to be carefully watched. This will include key drug-drug interactions.

Organ failure

Highlights any specific problems that may occur when using the drug in a particular organ failure.

Renal replacement therapy

Provides guidance on the effects of haemofiltration/dialysis on the handling of the drug. For some drugs, data are either limited or not available.

ABBREVIATIONS

ACE-I	angiotensin converting enzyme inhibitor
ACh	acetylcholine
ACT	activated clotting time
ADH	antidiuretic hormone
AF	atrial fibrillation
APTT	activated partial thromboplastin time
ARDS	acute respiratory distress syndrome
AUC	area under the curve
AV	atrioventricular
BP	blood pressure
CABG	coronary artery bypass graft
cAMP	cyclic AMP
CC	creatinine clearance
CMV	cytomegalovirus
CNS	central nervous system
CO	cardiac output
COPD	chronic obstructive pulmonary disease
CPR	cardiopulmonary resuscitation
CSF	cerebrospinal fluid
CT	computerised tomography
CVVH	continuous veno–venous haemofiltration
CVVHD	continuous veno–venous haemodiafiltration
DI	diabetes insipidus
DIC	disseminated intravascular coagulation
DVT	deep vein thrombosis
EBV	Epstein Barr virus
ECG	electrocardiogram
EEG	electroencephalogram
EMD	electromechanical dissociation
ESBL	extended-spectrum beta-lactamases
ETCO$_2$	end–tidal carbon dioxide concentration
FBC	full blood count
FFP	fresh frozen plasma
g	gram
GFR	glomerular filtration rate
GI	gastrointestinal
HD	haemodialysis
HOCM	hypertrophic obstructive cardiomyopathy
h	hour
HR	heart rate
ICP	intracranial pressure
ICU	intensive care unit
IHD	ischaemic heart disease
IM	intramuscular
INR	international normalised ratio
IOP	intraocular pressure

IPPV	intermittent positive pressure ventilation
IV	intravenous
K^+	potassium
kg	kilogram
l	litre
LFT	liver function tests
LMWH	low molecular weight heparin
MAOI	monoamine oxidase inhibitor
M6G	morphine-6-glucuronide
mg	milligram
MH	malignant hyperthermia
MI	myocardial infarction
MIC	minimum inhibitory concentration
min	minute
ml	millilitre
MRSA	meticillin-resistant *Staphylococcus aureus*
NG	nasogastric route
ng	nanogram
NIV	non-invasive ventilation
NJ	nasojejunal
nocte	at night
NSAID	non-steroidal anti-inflammatory drugs
PaCO$_2$	partial pressure of carbon dioxide in arterial blood
PaO$_2$	partial pressure of oxygen in arterial blood
PCA	patient controlled analgesia
PCP	*Pneumocystis carinii* pneumonia
PCWP	pulmonary capillary wedge pressure
PD	peritoneal dialysis
PE	pulmonary embolism
PEA	pulseless electrical activity
PEG	percutaneous endoscopic gastrostomy
PEJ	percutaneous endoscopic jejunostomy
PO	*per orum* (by mouth)
PPI	proton pump inhibitor
PR	*per rectum* (rectal route)
PRN	*pro re nata* (as required)
PT	prothrombin time
PVC	polyvinyl chloride
PVD	peripheral vascular disease
s	second
SC	subcutaneous
SIRS	systemic inflammatory response syndrome
SL	sublingual
SSRI	selective serotonin re-uptake inhibitors
STEMI	ST-segment elevation myocardial infarction
SVR	systemic vascular resistance
SVT	supraventricular tachycardia

TFT	thyroid function tests
TNF	tumour necrosis factor
TPN	total parenteral nutrition
U&E	urea and electrolytes
VF	ventricular fibrillation
VRE	vancomycin-resistant *Enterococcus faecium*
VT	ventricular tachycardia
WFI	water for injection
WPW syndrome	Wolff–Parkinson–White syndrome

ACKNOWLEDGEMENTS

I would like to thank the colleagues from whom I have sought advice during the preparation of this book. In particular, I acknowledge the assistance of Dr Daniel Weiand, Specialty Registrar in Microbiology, and Emily Waterman, Directorate Pharmacist for Critical Care. HP.

I would like to thank the staff of UCLH ICU for asking many searching questions about drug therapy, the answers to many of which fill these pages.

I would also like to acknowledge Keny Mole's UCLH Injectable Medicines Administration Guide.

RS.

ACKNOWLEDGEMENTS

Drugs:
An A–Z Guide

ACETAZOLAMIDE

Acetazolamide is a carbonic anhydrase inhibitor normally used to reduce intra-ocular pressure in glaucoma. Metabolic alkalosis may be partially corrected by the use of acetazolamide. The most common cause of metabolic alkalosis on the ICU is usually the result of furosemide administration.

Uses
Metabolic alkalosis (unlicensed)

Contraindications
Hypokalaemia
Hyponatraemia
Hyperchloraemic acidosis
Severe liver failure
Renal failure
Sulphonamide hypersensitivity

Administration
• IV: 250–500 mg, given over 3–5 min every 8 hours

Reconstitute with 5 ml WFI
Monitor: FBC, U&E and acid/base balance

How not to use acetazolamide
IM injection – painful
Not for prolonged use

Adverse effects
Metabolic acidosis
Electrolyte disturbances (hypokalaemia and hyponatraemia)
Blood disorders
Abnormal LFT

Cautions
Avoid extravasation at injection site (risk of necrosis)
Avoid prolonged use (risk of adverse effects)
Concurrent use with phenytoin ($\uparrow$ serum level of phenytoin)

Organ failure
Renal: avoid if possible (metabolic acidosis)

CC (ml/min)	Dose (mg)	Interval (h)
20–50	250	Up to 6
10–20	250	Up to 12
<10	250	24

Hepatic: avoid (abnormal LFT)

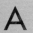

ACETYLCYSTEINE (Parvolex)

Acetylcysteine is an effective antidote to paracetamol if administered within 8 hours after an overdose. Although the protective effect diminishes progressively as the overdose–treatment interval increases, acetylcysteine can still be of benefit up to 24 hours after the overdose. In paracetamol overdose the hepatotoxicity is due to formation of a toxic metabolite. Hepatic reduced glutathione inactivates the toxic metabolite by conjugation, but glutathione stores are depleted with hepatotoxic doses of paracetamol. Acetylcysteine, being a sulphydryl (SH) group donor, protects the liver probably by restoring depleted hepatic reduced glutathione or by acting as an alternative substrate for the toxic metabolite.

Acetylcysteine may have significant cytoprotective effects. The cellular damage associated with sepsis, trauma, burns, pancreatitis, hepatic failure and tissue reperfusion following acute MI may be mediated by the formation and release of large quantities of free radicals that overwhelm and deplete endogenous antioxidants (e.g. glutathione). Acetylcysteine is a scavenger of oxygen free radicals. In addition, acetylcysteine is a glutathione precursor capable of replenishing depleted intracellular glutathione and, in theory, augmenting antioxidant defences (p. 288).

Acetylcysteine can be used to reduce the nephrotoxic effects of intravenous contrast media. Possible mechanisms include scavenging a variety of oxygen-derived free radicals and the improvement of endothelium-dependent vasodilation.

Nebulised acetylcysteine can be used as a mucolytic agent. It reduces sputum viscosity by disrupting the disulphide bonds in the mucus glycoproteins and enhances mucociliary clearance, thus facilitating easier expectoration.

Uses

Paracetamol overdose
Antioxidant (unlicensed)
Prevent IV contrast-induced nephropathy (unlicensed)
Reduce sputum viscosity and facilitate easier expectoration (unlicensed)
As a sulphydryl group donor to prevent the development of nitrate tolerance (unlicensed)

A

Administration

Paracetamol overdose

- IV infusion: 150 mg/kg in 200 ml glucose 5% over 60 min, followed by 50 mg/kg in 500 ml glucose 5% over 4 h, then 100 mg/kg in 1 litre glucose 5% over the next 16 h

Weight (kg)	Initial	Second	Third
	150 mg/kg in 200 ml glucose 5% over 60 min	50 mg/kg in 500 ml glucose 5% over 4 h	100 mg/kg in 1 litre glucose 5% over 16 h
	Parvolex (ml)	Parvolex (ml)	Parvolex (ml)
50	37.5	12.5	25
60	45.0	15.0	30
70	52.5	17.5	35
80	60.0	20.0	40
90	67.5	22.5	45
x	0.75x	0.25x	0.5x

For children >20 kg: same doses and regimen but in half the quantity of IV fluid

ACETYLCYSTEINE (Parvolex)

5

ACETYLCYSTEINE (Parvolex)

Treatment nomogram

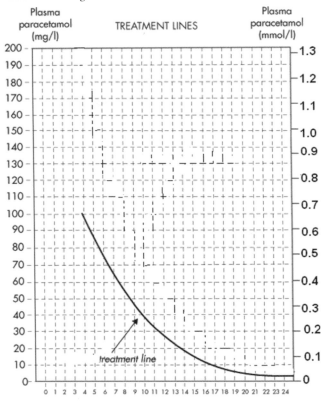

Hours after ingestion

Patients whose plasma concentrations fall on or above the treatment line should receive acetylcysteine. The prognostic value after 15 hours is uncertain, although a plasma-paracetamol concentration on or above the treatment line is likely to carry a serious risk of liver damage. Use acetylcysteine for paracetamol overdose irrespective of the plasma paracetamol level if the overdose is staggered or there is doubt over the time of paracetamol ingestion, or paracetamol overdose with a timed plasma paracetamol concentration on or above a single treatment line joining points of 100 mg/L at 4 hours and 15 mg/L at 15 hours regardless of risk factors of hepatotoxicity.

Antioxidant

- IV infusion: 75–100 mg/kg in 1 litre glucose 5%, give over 24 h (rate 40 ml/h)

Prevent IV contrast-induced nephropathy (not required for oral/enterally administered contrast)

- IV bolus 1200 mg pre-contrast, then after 12 hours 1200 mg PO/NG (or IV if nil-by-mouth) 12 hourly for 48 hours (there is also evidence for 600 mg as an alternate dose)

Dilution: make up to 20 ml with glucose 5%

To be given in conjunction with IV sodium bicarbonate 1.26% at 3 ml/kg/hr over 1 hour prior to IV contrast. Continue at reduced rate of 1 mg/kg/hr for 6 hours following contrast

Reduce sputum viscosity

- Nebulised: 4 ml (800 mg) undiluted Parvolex (20%) driven by air, 8 hourly

Administer before chest physiotherapy

How not to use acetylcysteine
Do not drive nebuliser with oxygen (oxygen inactivates acetylcysteine)

Adverse effects
Anaphylactoid reactions (nausea, vomiting, flushing, itching, rashes, bronchospasm, hypotension)
Fluid overload

Cautions
There are no contraindications to treatment of paracetamol overdose with acetylcysteine
Asthmatics (risk of bronchospasm)
Pulmonary oedema (worsens)
Each 10 ml ampoule contains Na^+ 12.8 mmol ($\uparrow$ total body sodium)

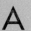

ACICLOVIR (Zovirax)

Interferes with herpes virus DNA polymerase, inhibiting viral DNA replication. Aciclovir is renally excreted and has a prolonged half-life in renal impairment.

Uses
Herpes simplex virus infections:

- HSV encephalitis
- HSV genital, labial, peri-anal and rectal infections

Varicella zoster virus infections:

- Beneficial in the immunocompromised patients when given IV within 72 hours: prevents complications of pneumonitis, hepatitis or thrombocytopenia
- In patients with normal immunity, may be considered if the oph-thalmic branch of the trigeminal nerve is involved

Contraindications
Not suitable for CMV or EBV infections

Administration
- IV: 5–10 mg/kg 8 hourly (i.e. 5 mg/kg for herpes simplex, herpes zoster; 10 mg/kg for herpes zoster in immunocompromised, herpes simplex encephalitis

Available in 250 mg/10 ml and 500 mg/20 ml ready-diluted or in 250 mg and 500 mg vials for reconstitution
Reconstitute 250 mg vial with 10 ml WFI or sodium chloride 0.9% (25 mg/ml)
Reconstitute 500 mg vial with 20 ml WFI or sodium chloride 0.9% (25 mg/ml)
Take the reconstituted solution (25 mg/ml) and make up to 50 ml (for 250 mg vial) or 100 ml (for 500 mg vial) with sodium chloride 0.9% or glucose 5%, and give over 1 hour

Ensure patient is well hydrated before treatment is administered

If fluid-restricted, can give centrally via syringe pump undiluted (unlicensed)

In renal impairment:

CC (ml/min)	Dose (mg/kg)	Interval (h)
25–50	5–10	12
10–25	5–10	24
<10	2.5–5	24

How not to use aciclovir
Rapid IV infusion (precipitation of drug in renal tubules leading to renal impairment)

Adverse effects
Phlebitis
Reversible renal failure
Elevated liver function tests
CNS toxicity (tremors, confusion and fits)

Cautions
Concurrent use of methotrexate
Renal impairment (reduce dose)
Dehydration/hypovolaemia (renal impairment due to precipitation in renal tubules)

Renal replacement therapy
CVVH dose dependent on clearance rate as described in Short Notes Renal Replacement Therapy (p. 300–303) and CC table given previously. Not significantly cleared by PD or HD, dose as if CC <10 ml/min, i.e. 2.5–5 mg/kg IV every 24 hours. The dose is dependent upon the indication.

A

ACICLOVIR (Zovirax)

ADENOSINE (Adenocor)

This endogenous nucleoside is safe and effective in ending >90% of re-entrant paroxysmal SVT. However, this is not the most common type of SVT in the critically ill patient. After an IV bolus effects are immediate (10–30 seconds), dose-related and transient (half-life <10 seconds; entirely eliminated from plasma in <1 minute, being degraded by vascular endothelium and erythrocytes). Its elimination is not affected by renal/hepatic disease. Adenosine works faster and is superior to verapamil. It may be used in cardiac failure, in hypotension and with β-blockers, in all of which verapamil is contraindicated.

Uses
It has both therapeutic and diagnostic uses:

- Alternative to DC cardioversion in terminating paroxysmal SVT, including those associated with WPW syndrome
- Determining the origin of broad complex tachycardia; SVT responds, VT does not (predictive accuracy 92%; partly because VT may occasionally respond). Though adenosine does no harm in VT, verapamil may produce hypotension or cardiac arrest

Contraindications
Second- or third-degree heart block (unless pacemaker fitted)
Sick sinus syndrome (unless pacemaker fitted)
Asthmatic – may cause bronchospasm
Patients on dipyridamole (drastically prolongs the half-life and enhances the effects of adenosine – may lead to dangerously prolonged high-degree AV block)

Administration

- Rapid IV bolus: 3 mg over 1–2 seconds into a large vein, followed by rapid flushing with sodium chloride 0.9%

  If no effect within 2 min, give 6 mg
  If no effect within 2 min, give 12 mg
  If no effect, abandon adenosine
  Need continuous ECG monitoring
  More effective given via a central vein or into right atrium

How not to use adenosine
Without continuous ECG monitor

Adverse effects
Flushing (18%), dyspnoea (12%) and chest discomfort are the commonest side-effects but are well tolerated and invariably last <1 min. If given to an asthmatic and bronchospasm occurs, this may last up to 30 min (use aminophylline to reverse).

Cautions

AF or atrial flutter with accessory pathway (↑ conduction down anomalous pathway may increase)

Early relapse of paroxysmal SVT is more common than with verapamil but usually responds to further doses

Adenosine's effect is enhanced and extended by dipyridamole – if essential to give with dipyridamole, reduce initial dose to 0.5–1 mg

A

ADENOSINE (Adenocor)

ADRENALINE

Both α- and β-adrenergic receptors are stimulated. Low doses tend to produce predominantly β-effects while higher doses tend to produce predominantly α-effects. Stimulation of β_1-receptors in the heart increases the rate and force of contraction, resulting in an increase in cardiac output. Stimulation of α_1-receptor causes peripheral vasoconstriction, which increases the systolic BP. Stimulation of β_2-receptors causes bronchodilatation and vasodilatation in certain vascular beds (skeletal muscles). Consequently, total systemic resistance may actually fall, explaining the decrease in diastolic BP that is sometimes seen.

Uses
Low cardiac output states
Bronchospasm
Cardiac arrest (p. 257)
Anaphylaxis (p. 259)

Contraindications
Before adequate intravascular volume replacement

Administration
Low cardiac output states
Dose: $0.01-0.30\,\mu g/kg/min$ IV infusion via a central vein
Titrate dose according to HR, BP, cardiac output, presence of ectopic beats and urine output
4 mg made up to 50 ml glucose 5%

Dosage chart (ml/h)

Weight (kg)	Dose (µg/kg/min)				
	0.02	0.05	0.1	0.15	0.2
50	0.8	1.9	3.8	5.6	7.5
60	0.9	2.3	4.5	6.8	9.0
70	1.1	2.6	5.3	7.9	10.5
80	1.2	3.0	6.0	9.0	12
90	1.4	3.4	6.8	10.1	13.5
100	1.5	3.8	7.5	11.3	15.0
110	1.7	4.1	8.3	12.4	16.5
120	1.8	4.5	9.0	13.5	18.0

Bronchospasm

- 0.5–1 mg nebulised PRN
- 0.5–1 ml of 1:1000 (0.5–1 mg) made up to 5 ml with sodium chloride 0.9%

Cardiac arrest (p. 257)

- IV bolus: 10 ml 1 in 10 000 solution (1 mg)

Anaphylaxis (p. 259)

- IV bolus: 0.5–1.0 ml 1 in 10 000 solution (50–100 μg), may be repeated PRN, according to BP

How not to use adrenaline
In the absence of haemodynamic monitoring
Do not connect to CVP lumen used for monitoring pressure (surge of drug during flushing of line)
Incompatible with alkaline solutions, e.g. sodium bicarbonate, furosemide, phenytoin and enoximone

Adverse effects
Arrhythmia
Tachycardia
Hypertension
Myocardial ischaemia
Increased lactate levels

Cautions
Acute myocardial ischaemia or MI

A

ADRENALINE

13

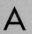

ALFENTANIL

It is an opioid 30 times more potent than morphine and its duration is shorter than that of fentanyl. The maximum effect occurs about 1 min after IV injection. Duration of action following an IV bolus is between 5 and 10 min. Its distribution volume and lipophilicity are lower than fentanyl. It is ideal for infusion and may be the agent of choice in renal failure. The context-sensitive half-life may be prolonged following IV infusion. In patients with hepatic failure the elimination half-life may be markedly increased and a prolonged duration of action may be seen.

Uses
Patients receiving short-term ventilation

Contraindications
Airway obstruction
Concomitant use of MAOI

Administration
- IV bolus: 500 µg every 10 min as necessary
- IV infusion rate: 1–5 mg/h (up to 1 µg/kg/min)

Draw ampoules up neat to make infusion, i.e. 0.5 mg/ml or dilute to a convenient volume with glucose 5% or sodium chloride 0.9%

How not to use alfentanil
In combination with an opioid partial agonist, e.g. buprenorphine (antagonizes opioid effects)

Adverse effects
Respiratory depression and apnoea
Bradycardia
Nausea and vomiting
Delayed gastric emptying
Reduce intestinal mobility
Biliary spasm
Constipation
Urinary retention
Chest wall rigidity (may interfere with ventilation)

A

Cautions

Enhanced sedative and respiratory depression from interaction with:

- benzodiazepines
- antidepressants
- anti–psychotics

Avoid concomitant use of and for 2 weeks after MAOI discontinued (risk of CNS excitation or depression – hypertension, hyperpyrexia, convulsions and coma)

Head injury and neurosurgical patients (may exacerbate ↑ ICP as a result of ↑ $PaCO_2$)
Erythromycin (↓ clearance of alfentanil)

Organ failure

Respiratory: ↑ respiratory depression
Hepatic: enhanced and prolonged sedative effect

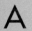

ALTEPLASE (Actilyse)

The use of thrombolytics is well established in myocardial infarction and pulmonary embolism. They act by activating plasminogen to form plasmin, which degrades fibrin and so breaks up thrombi. Alteplase or tissue-type plasminogen activator (rt-PA) can be used in major pulmonary embolism associated with hypoxia and haemodynamic compromise. Whilst alteplase is more expensive than streptokinase, it is the preferred thrombolytic as it does not worsen hypotension. Severe bleeding is a potential adverse effect of alteplase and requires discontinuation of the thrombolytic and may require administration of coagulation factors and antifibrinolytic drugs (such as tranexamic acid).

Uses
Major pulmonary embolism
Acute myocardial infarction
Acute stroke

Contraindications
Recent haemorrhage, trauma or surgery
Coagulation defects
Severe hypertension
Oesophageal varices
Severe liver disease
Acute pancreatitis

Administration
- Pulmonary embolism

  Ideally, APTT ratio should be <1.5 before thrombolysis starts, but do not delay if condition appears to be immediately life-threatening. IV alteplase: for stable massive PE patients, give 10 mg IV bolus over 1–2 mins, then 90 mg over 2 hours (max. total dose 1.5 mg/kg if <65 kg)

  For patients who are rapidly deteriorating and in whom cardiac arrest is imminent, or who have an inhouse cardiac arrest, give 50 mg IV bolus alteplase and reassess at 30 mins

  Restart unfractionated heparin approximately 2.5 hours after the end of the alteplase infusion, urgently checking that APTT ratio is <2 before doing so. If APTT ratio is <1.5, give an IV bolus of 5,000 units (or 70–100 units/kg for small adults), followed by IV infusion to keep APTT ratio between 1.5 and 2.5. If APTT ratio is >1.5, start heparin infusion without a bolus. Start warfarin on day 3 to 7 of heparin therapy and continue until INR in range for 2 consecutive days with not less than 5 days overlap

A

Dissolve in WFI to a concentration of 1 mg/ml (50–mg vial with 50 ml WFI). Foaming may occur; this will dissipate after standing for a few minutes

Monitor: BP (treat if systolic BP >180 mmHg or diastolic BP >105 mmHg)

• Myocardial infarction

Accelerated regimen (initiated within 6 hours of symptom onset), 15 mg IV, then 50 mg IV infusion over 30 min, then 35 mg over 60 min (total dose 100 mg over 90 min); in patients <65 kg, 15 mg by IV, the IV infusion of 0.75 mg/kg over 30 min, then 0.5 mg/kg over 60 min (max. total dose 100 mg over 90 min)

Myocardial infarction, initiated within 6–12 hours of symptom onset, 10 mg IV, followed by IV infusion of 50 mg over 60 min, then 4 infusions each of 10 mg over 30 min (total dose 100 mg over 3 hours; max. 1.5 mg/kg in patients <65 kg)

• Acute stroke

Treatment must begin within 3 hours of symptom onset.
IV: 900 μg/kg (max. 90 mg), initial 10% of dose by IV injection over 3 min, remainder by IV infusion over 60 min
Not recommended in the elderly over 80 years of age

Management of bleeding and thrombolysis
Bleeding may occur even when coagulation screening tests are normal. Monitor regularly for clinical signs of bleeding. If internal bleeding suspected, consider whether the infusion of thrombolytic therapy should be stopped and investigations undertaken. If bleeding is local and minor, apply sustained local pressure. For more serious bleeding, stop the infusion of thrombolytic therapy and heparin (restore depleted fibrinogen, factors V and VIII within 12–24 hours). For severe, life-threatening bleeding, discontinue thrombolytic therapy and heparin. Administer IV aprotinin immediately, (500,000–1,000,000 KIU (50–100 ml, consider patient's weight) over 10–20 minutes, then an IV infusion of 200,000–500,000 KIU per hour (20–50 ml/h) until bleeding stops. Alternatively, administer tranexamic acid IV 1 g over 15 minutes, repeated 8 hourly as necessary. Administer FFP and/or cryoprecipitate to replenish depleted clotting factors, depending on coagulation screen. Red cells should be infused as clinically indicated. For life-threatening haematoma (e.g. intracranial) consider measures either to evacuate or relieve pressure.

ALTEPLASE (Actilyse)

17

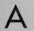

How not to use alteplase
Not to be infused in glucose solution

Adverse effects
Nausea and vomiting
Bleeding

Cautions
Acute stroke (risk of cerebral bleed)
Diabetic retinopathy (risk of retinal bleeding)
Abdominal aortic aneurysm and enlarged left atrium with AF (risk of embolisation)

Organ failure
Renal: risk of hyperkalaemia
Hepatic: avoid in severe liver failure
Acknowledgement: UCLH Foundation Trust PE Guideline

AMINOPHYLLINE

The ethylenediamine salt of theophylline. It is a non-specific inhibitor of phosphodiesterase, producing increased levels of cAMP. Increased cAMP levels result in:

- Bronchodilation
- CNS stimulation
- Positive inotropic and chronotropic effects
- Diuresis

Theophylline has been claimed to reduce fatigue of diaphragmatic muscles

Uses
Prevention and treatment of bronchospasm

Contraindications
Uncontrolled arrhythmias
Hyperthyroidism

Administration

- Loading dose: 5 mg/kg IV, diluted in 100 ml sodium chloride 0.9% or glucose 5%, given over 30 min, followed by maintenance dose 0.1–0.8 mg/kg/h

Dilute 500 mg (20 ml) aminophylline (25 mg/ml) in 480 ml sodium chloride 9% or glucose 5% to give a concentration of 1 mg/ml
No loading dose if already on oral theophylline preparations (toxicity)
Reduce maintenance dose (0.1–0.3 mg/kg/h) in the elderly and patients with congestive heart failure and liver disease
Increase maintenance dose (0.8–1 mg/kg/h) in children (6 months–16 years) and young adult smokers
Monitor plasma level (p. 250)
Therapeutic range 55–110 mmol/l or 10–20 mg/l
The injection can be administered nasogastrically (unlicensed). This may be useful as there is no liquid preparation of aminophylline or theophylline. To convert from IV to NG, keep the total daily dose the same, but divide into four equal doses. Aminophylline modified-release tablets are taken by mouth twice daily. Alternatively, if these are crushed up to go down a nasogastric tube then they will lose their slow-release characteristic and will need to be administered four times per day keeping the total daily dose the same

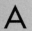

Dosage chart: ml/h

Weight: kg	Dose: mg/kg/h									
	0.1	0.2	0.3	0.4	0.5	0.6	0.7	0.8	0.9	1
50	5	10	15	20	25	30	35	40	45	50
60	6	12	18	24	30	36	42	48	54	60
70	7	14	21	28	35	42	49	56	63	70
80	8	16	24	32	40	48	56	64	72	80
90	9	18	27	36	45	54	63	72	81	90
100	10	20	30	40	50	60	70	80	90	100
110	11	22	33	44	55	66	77	88	99	110
120	12	24	36	48	60	72	84	96	108	120
	• Elderly • Congestive Heart failure • Liver disease			• Usual adult maintenance				• Children • Young adult smokers		

How not to use aminophylline
Rapid IV administration (hypotension, arrhythmias)

Adverse effects
Tachycardia
Arrhythmias
Convulsions

Cautions
Subject to enzyme inducers and inhibitors (p. 248)
Concurrent use of erythromycin and ciprofloxacin: reduce dose

Organ failure
Cardiac: prolonged half-life (reduce dose)
Hepatic: prolonged half-life (reduce dose)

AMIODARONE

A

Amiodarone has a broad spectrum of activity on the heart. In addition to having an anti-arrhythmic activity, it also has anti-anginal effects. This may result from its α- and β-adrenoceptor-blocking properties as well as from its calcium channel-blocking effect in the coronary vessels. It causes minimal myocardial depression. It is therefore often a first-line drug in critical care situations. It has an extremely long half-life (15–105 days). Unlike oral amiodarone, IV administration usually acts relatively rapidly (20–30 min). Oral bioavailability is 50%, therefore 600 mg PO/NG is equivalent to 300 mg IV. Overlap the initial oral and IV therapy for 16 to 24 hours. An oral loading dose regimen is necessary even when the patient has been adequately 'loaded' intravenously. This is because amiodarone has a large volume of distribution (4000 l) and a long half-life. The high initial plasma levels quickly dissipate as the drug binds to the peripheral lipophilic tissues. Thus a prolonged loading regimen is required. When the cause of the arrhythmia has resolved, e.g. sepsis, then amiodarone treatment can be stopped abruptly.

Uses
Good results with both ventricular and supraventricular arrhythmias, including those associated with WPW syndrome.

Contraindications
Iodine sensitivity (amiodarone contains iodine)
Sinus bradycardia (risk of asystole)
Heart block (unless pacemaker fitted)

Administration
- Loading: 300 mg in 25–250 ml glucose 5% IV over 20–120 min, followed by 900 mg in 50–500 ml glucose 5% over 24 hours. If fluid-restricted, up to 900 mg can be diluted in 50 ml glucose 5% and administered centrally
- Maintenance: 600 mg IV daily for 7 days, then 400 mg IV daily for 7 days, then 200 mg IV daily

Administer IV via central line. A volumetric pump should be used as the droplet size of amiodarone may be reduced.
Continuous cardiac monitoring

- Oral: 200 mg 8 hourly for 7 days, then 200 mg 12 hourly for 7 days, then 200 mg daily

How not to use amiodarone
Incompatible with sodium chloride 0.9%
Do not use via peripheral vein (thrombophlebitis)

AMIODARONE

Adverse effects

Short-term
Skin reactions common
Vasodilation and hypotension or bradycardia after rapid infusion
Corneal microdeposits (reversible on stopping)

Long-term
Pulmonary fibrosis, alveolitis and pneumonitis (usually reversible on stopping)
Liver dysfunction (asymptomatic ↑ in LFT common)
Hypo- or hyperthyroidism (check TFT before starting drug)
Peripheral neuropathy, myopathy and cerebellar dysfunction (reversible on stopping)

Cautions
Increased risk of bradycardia, AV block and myocardial depression with β-blockers and calcium-channel antagonists

Potentiates the effect of digoxin, theophylline and warfarin – reduce dose

Organ failure
Hepatic: worsens
Renal: accumulation of iodine may ↑ risk of thyroid dysfunction

AMITRIPTYLINE

A tricyclic antidepressant with sedative properties. When given at night it will help to promote sleep. It may take up to 4 weeks before any beneficial antidepressant effect is seen. It is used less often now in depression due to the high rate of fatality in overdose.

Uses
Depression in patients requiring long-term ICU stay, particularly where sedation is required
Difficulty with sleep
Neuropathic pain (unlicensed indication)

Contraindications
Recent myocardial infarction
Arrhythmia
Heart block
Severe liver disease

Administration
- Oral: depression 25–75 mg nocte

  Neuropathic pain 10–25 mg at night, increased if necessary up to 75 mg daily

How not to use amitriptyline
During the daytime (disturbs the normal sleep pattern)

Adverse effects
Antimuscarinic effects (dry mouth, blurred vision, urinary retention)
Arrhythmias
Postural hypotension
Confusion
Hyponatraemia

Cautions
Cardiac disease (risk of arrhythmias)
Hepatic failure
Acute angle glaucoma
Avoid long-term use if patient represents a suicide risk
Concurrent use of MAOI
Additive CNS depression with other sedative agents
May potentiate direct-acting sympathomimetic drugs
Prostatic hypertrophy–urinary retention (unless patient's bladder catheterized)

Organ failure
CNS: sedative effects increased
Hepatic: sedative effects increased

AMPHOTERICIN (Fungizone)

Amphotericin is active against most fungi and yeasts. It also has useful activity against protozoa, including *Leishmania* spp., *Naeglaria* and *Hartmanella*. It is not absorbed from the gut when given orally. When given IV it is highly toxic and side-effects are common. The liposomal formulation is less toxic, particularly in terms of nephrotoxicity.

Uses
Suppress gut carriage of *Candida* species by the oral route
Severe systemic fungal infections:
    Aspergillosis
    Candidiasis
    Coccidiomycosis
    Cryptococcosis
    Histoplasmosis

Administration
- Oral: suppression of gut carriage of *Candida*

  100–200 mg 6 hourly

- IV: systemic fungal infections

  Initial test dose of 1 mg given over 30 min, then 250 µg/kg daily, gradually increased if tolerated to 1 mg/kg daily over 4 days

- For severe infection: 1 mg/kg daily or 1.5 mg/kg daily on alternate days

  Available in 20-ml vial containing 50 mg amphotericin
  Reconstitute with 10 ml WFI (5 mg/ml). Add phosphate buffer to the glucose 5% bag before amphotericin is added. The phosphate buffer label will state the volume to be added; then further dilute the reconstituted solution as follows:

For peripheral administration:
    Dilute further with 500 ml glucose 5% (to 0.2 mg/ml)
    Give over 6 hours

For central administration:
    Dilute further with 50–100 ml glucose 5%
    Give over 6 hours

Prolonged treatment usually needed (duration depends on severity and nature of infection)

Monitor:
Serum potassium, magnesium and creatinine
FBC
LFT

A

How not to use amphotericin
Must not be given by rapid IV infusion (arrhythmias)
Not compatible with sodium chloride
There are two formulations of IV amphotericin and they are not interchangeable. Errors of this sort have caused lethal consequences or subtherapeutic doses

Adverse effects
Fever and rigors – common in first week. May need paracetamol, chlorphenamine and hydrocortisone premedication
Nephrotoxicity – major limiting toxicity. Usually reversible
Hypokalaemia/hypomagnesaemia – 25% will need supplements
Anaemia (normochromic, normocytic) – 75%. Due to bone marrow suppression
Cardiotoxicity – arrhythmias and hypotension with rapid IV bolus
Phlebitis – frequent change of injection site
Pulmonary reactions
GI upset – anorexia, nausea, vomiting

Cautions
Kidney disease
Concurrent use of other nephrotoxic drugs
Hypokalaemia – increased digoxin toxicity
Avoid concurrent administration of corticosteroids (except to treat febrile and anaphylactic reactions)

Organ failure
Renal: use only if no alternative; nephrotoxicity may be reduced with use of Amphocil or AmBisome

Renal replacement therapy
No further dose modification is required during renal replacement therapy

AMPHOTERICIN (Fungizone)

AMPHOTERICIN (LIPOSOMAL) – AmBisome

Amphotericin is active against most fungi and yeasts. It also has useful activity against protozoa, including *Leishmania* spp., *Naeglaria* and *Hartmanella*. AmBisome is a formulation of amphotericin encapsulated in liposomes. This renders the drug less toxic to the kidney than the parent compound. Each vial contains 50 mg amphotericin.

Uses
Severe systemic fungal infections, when conventional amphotericin is contraindicated because of toxicity, especially nephrotoxicity, or as a safer alternative to conventional amphotericin.

Administration
- IV: initially 1 mg/kg daily, ↑ if necessary to 3 mg/kg daily

Add 12 ml WFI to each 50-mg vial of liposomal amphotericin (4 mg/ml) Shake vigorously for at least 15 seconds

Calculate the amount of the 4 mg/ml solution required, i.e.:

    100 mg = 25 ml
    150 mg = 37.5 ml
    200 mg = 50 ml
    300 mg = 75 ml

Using the 5 micron filter provided add the required volume of the 4 mg/ml solution to at least equal volume of glucose 5% (final concentration 2 mg/ml) and given over 30–60 min

Although anaphylactic reactions are rare, before starting treatment an initial test dose of 1 mg should be given over 10 min, infusion stopped and patient observed for 30 min. Continue infusion if no signs of anaphylactic reaction

The diluted solution is stable for 24 hours

Monitor: serum potassium and magnesium

In renal dialysis patients, give AmBisome at the end of each dialysis

Although nephrotoxic, no dose adjustment is required in haemofiltration

How not to use liposomal amphotericin
Must not be given by rapid IV infusion (arrhythmias)

Not compatible with sodium chloride

Do not mix with other drugs

There are two formulations of IV amphotericin and they are not interchangeable. Errors of this sort have caused lethal consequences or subtherapeutic doses

Adverse effects
Prevalence and severity lower than conventional amphotericin

Cautions
Kidney disease
Concurrent use of nephrotoxic drugs
Avoid concurrent administration of corticosteroids (except to treat febrile and anaphylactic reactions)
Diabetic patient: each vial contains 900 mg sucrose

AMPHOTERICIN (LIPOSOMAL) – AmBisome

AMPICILLIN

Ampicillin has a spectrum of activity, which includes staphylococci, streptococci, most enterococci, *Listeria monocytogenes* and Gram −ve rods such as *Salmonella* spp., *Shigella* spp., *E. coli*, *H. influenzae* and *Proteus* spp. It is not active against *Pseudomonas aeruginosa* and *Klebsiella spp*. However due to acquired resistance almost all staphylococci, 50% of *E. coli* and up to 15% of *H. influenzae strains* are now resistant. All penicillin-resistant pneumococci and enterococci have reduced susceptibility to ampicillin. Amoxicillin is similar but better absorbed orally.

Uses
Urinary tract infections
Respiratory tract infections
Invasive salmonellosis
Serious infections with *Listeria monocytogenes*, including meningitis

Contraindications
Penicillin hypersensitivity

Administration
- IV: 500 mg–1 g diluted in 10 ml WFI, 4–6 hourly over 3–5 min
- Meningitis caused by *Listeria monocytogenes* (with gentamicin)

IV: 2 g diluted in 10 ml WFI every 4 hours over 3–5 minutes. Treat for 10–14 days

In renal impairment:

CC (ml/min)	Dose (g) depending on severity of infection	Interval (h)
10–20	500 mg–2	6
<10	250 mg–1	6

How not to use ampicillin
Not for intrathecal use (encephalopathy)
Do not mix in the same syringe with an aminoglycoside (efficacy of aminoglycoside reduced)

Adverse effects
Hypersensitivity
Skin rash increases in patients with infectious mononucleosis (90%), chronic lymphocytic leukaemia and HIV infections (discontinue drug)

A

Cautions
Severe renal impairment (reduce dose, rashes more common)

Renal replacement therapy
CVVH dose dependent on clearance rate as described in Short Notes Renal Replacement Therapy (p. 300–303) and CC table given previously
Not significantly cleared by PD or HD, dose as if CC <10 ml/min, i.e. 250 mg–1 g every 6 hours

AMPICILLIN

ANIDULAFUNGIN (Ecalta)

Anidulafungin (Ecalta) is an echinocandin, similar to caspofungin and micafungin. It covers a wide range of *Candida* species causing invasive candidiasis (including *C. krusei* and *C. glabrata*) and is eliminated by nonenzymatic degradation to an inactive metabolite. The key distinguishing features compared to caspofungin are simplicity of dosing regimen, storage at room temperature, narrower clinical indication and fewer drug interactions.

Uses
Invasive candidiasis in adult non-neutropenic patients

Contraindications
Hypersensitivity to echinocandin

Administration
- IV: Load with 200 mg on day 1, followed by 100 mg daily thereafter for a minimum of 14 days

  Reconstitute each vial with 30 ml solvent provided, allowing up to 5 min for reconstitution. Add the reconstituted solution to a bag of sodium chloride 0.9% or glucose 5%, i.e. 100 mg in 250 ml and 200 mg in 500 ml. Administer at 3 ml/min
  Available in vials containing 100 mg with solvent containing ethanol anhydrous in WFI

How not to use anidulafungin
Do not use in children under 18 years as insufficient data

Adverse effects
Coagulopathy
Convulsion
Headache
Increased creatinine
Hypokalaemia
Elevated LFT
Flushing
Diarrhoea, nausea and vomiting
Rash
Pruritus

Cautions
Hepatic failure worsening LFTs
The diluent contains the equivalent of 6 g of ethanol/100 mg of anidulafungin. Caution in breast feeding and pregnancy and high-risk groups, e.g. liver disease, epilepsy, alcoholism
Fructose intolerance

Organ failure
Renal: no dose adjustment necessary, as negligible renal clearance
Hepatic: no dose adjustment, as not metabolised in liver

Renal replacement therapy
Unlikely to be removed by dialysis, therefore no dose adjustment
required

A

ANIDULAFUNGIN (Ecalta)

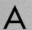

ATRACURIUM

Atracurium is a non-depolarising neuromuscular blocker that is broken down by Hofmann degradation and ester hydrolysis. The ampoules have to be stored in the fridge to prevent spontaneous degradation. Atracurium has an elimination half-life of 20 min. The principal metabolite is laudanosine, which can cause convulsions in dogs. Even with long-term infusions, the concentration of laudanosine is well below the seizure threshold (17 μg/ml). It is the agent of choice in renal and hepatic failure.

Uses
Muscle paralysis

Contraindications
Airway obstruction
To facilitate tracheal intubation in patients at risk of regurgitation

Administration
- IV bolus: 0.5 mg/kg, repeat with 0.15 mg/kg at 20–45 min interval
- IV infusion: 0.2–0.4 mg/kg/h

Monitor with peripheral nerve stimulator

How not to use atracurium
As part of a rapid sequence induction
In the conscious patient
By persons not trained to intubate trachea

Adverse effects
Bradycardia
Hypotension

Cautions
Asthmatics (histamine release)
Breathing circuit (disconnection)
Prolonged use (disuse muscle atrophy)

Organ failure
Hepatic: increased concentration of laudanosine
Renal: increased concentration of laudanosine

ATROPINE

The influence of atropine is most noticeable in healthy young adults in whom vagal tone is considerable. In infancy and old age, even large doses may fail to accelerate the heart.

Uses
Asystole (p. 257)
EMD or PEA with ventricular rate <60/min (p. 257)
Sinus bradycardia – will increase BP as a result
Reversal of muscarinic effects of anticholinesterases (neostigmine)
Organophosphate poisoning
Hypersalivation

Contraindications
Complete heart block
Tachycardia

Administration
- Bradycardia: 0.3–1 mg IV bolus, up to 3 mg (total vagolytic dose), may be diluted with WFI
- Asystole: 3 mg IV bolus, once only (p. 257)
- EMD or PEA with ventricular rate <60/min: 3 mg IV bolus, once only (p. 257)
- Reversal of muscarinic effects of anticholinesterase: 1.2 mg for every 2.5 mg neostigmine
- Organophosphate poisoning: 1–2 mg initially, then further 1–2 mg every 30 min PRN
- Hypersalivation sublingual 1% atropine eye drops 1 drop twice daily (unlicensed indication) – can cause hallucinations

How not to use atropine
Slow IV injection of doses <0.3 mg (bradycardia caused by medullary vagal stimulation)

Adverse effects
Drowsiness, confusion
Dry mouth
Blurred vision
Urinary retention
Tachycardia
Pyrexia (suppression of sweating)
Atrial arrhythmias and atrioventricular dissociation (without significant cardiovascular symptoms)
Dose >5 mg results in restlessness and excitation, hallucinations, delirium and coma

Cautions

Elderly (↑ CNS side-effects)

Child with pyrexia (further ↑ temperature)

Acute myocardial ischaemia or MI (tachycardia may cause worsening)

Prostatic hypertrophy–urinary retention (unless patient's bladder catheterised)

Paradoxically, bradycardia may occur at low doses (<0.3 mg)

Acute-angle glaucoma (further ↑ IOP)

Pregnancy (foetal tachycardia)

BENZYLPENICILLIN

Benzylpenicillin can only be given parenterally. It is active against most streptococci but the majority of strains of *Staphylococcus aureus* are resistant due to penicillinase production. Resistance rates are increasing in *Streptococcus pneumoniae*, and benzylpenicillin should probably not be used for empiric treatment of meningitis unless local levels of resistance are extremely low. All strains of *Neisseria meningitidis* remain sensitive.

Uses
- Infective endocarditis
- Streptococcal infections including severe necrotising soft tissue infections and severe pharyngeal infections
- Pneumococcal infections – excluding empiric therapy of meningitis
- Gas gangrene and prophylaxis in limb amputation
- Meningococcal meningitis with sensitive organism
- Tetanus
- Post-splenectomy prophylaxis

Contraindications
Penicillin hypersensitivity

Administration
IV: 600–1200 mg diluted in 10 ml WFI, 6 hourly over 3–5 min, higher doses should be given for severe infections in 100 ml of glucose 5% or sodium chloride 0.9% and given over 30–60 min
Infective endocarditis: 7.2 g/24 h (with gentamicin)
Adult meningitis: 14.4 g/24 h
Post-splenectomy prophylaxis: 600 mg 12 hourly
Give at a rate not >300 mg/min

In renal impairment:

CC (ml/min)	Dose (range depending on severity of infection)
10–20	600 mg–2.4 g every 6 hours
<10	600 mg–1.2 g every 6 hours

How not to use benzylpenicillin
Not for intrathecal use (encephalopathy)
Do not mix in the same syringe with an aminoglycoside (efficacy of aminoglycoside reduced)

B

Adverse effects
Hypersensitivity
Haemolytic anaemia
Transient neutropenia and thrombocytopenia
Convulsions (high-dose or renal failure)

Cautions
Anaphylactic reactions frequent (1:100 000)
Severe renal impairment (reduce dose, high doses may cause convulsions)

Renal replacement therapy
CVVH dose dependent on clearance rate as described in Short Notes Renal Replacement Therapy (p. 300–303) and CC table given previously. Not significantly cleared by PD or HD, dose as if CC < 10 ml/min (600 mg–2.4 g every 6 hours depending on severity of infection)

BUMETANIDE

B

A loop diuretic similar to furosemide but 40 times more potent. Ototoxicity may be less with bumetanide than with furosemide, but nephrotoxicity may be worse.

Uses
Acute oliguric renal failure
May convert acute oliguric to non-oliguric renal failure. Other measures must be taken to ensure adequate circulating blood volume and renal perfusion pressure
Pulmonary oedema secondary to acute left ventricular failure
Oedema associated with congestive cardiac failure, hepatic failure and renal disease

Contraindications
Oliguria secondary to hypovolaemia

Administration
- IV bolus: 1–2 mg 1–2 min, repeat in 2–3 h if needed
- IV infusion: 2–5 mg in 100 ml glucose 5% or sodium chloride 0.9% saline, given over 30–60 min

Adverse effects
Hyponatraemia, hypokalaemia, hypomagnesaemia
Hyperuricaemia, hyperglycaemia
Hypovolaemia
Ototoxicity
Nephrotoxicity
Pancreatitis

Cautions
Amphotericin (increased risk of hypokalaemia)
Aminoglycosides (increased nephrotoxicity and ototoxicity)
Digoxin toxicity (due to hypokalaemia)

Organ failure
Renal: may need to increase dose for effect

Renal replacement therapy
No further dose modification is required during renal replacement therapy

CARBOCISTEINE (Mucodyne)

Carbocisteine affects the nature and amount of mucus glycoprotein that is secreted by the respiratory tract. It is a well-tolerated treatment with a favourable safety profile that provides symptomatic relief to some patients with sputum production in COPD. It can be used in the ICU to treat mucous plugging as an alternative to saline or acetyl-cysteine nebulisation. In addition to its mucoregulatory activity, carbocisteine exhibits free-radical scavenging and anti-inflammatory properties. There is a theoretical risk of gastric erosion because carbocisteine may disrupt the gastric mucosal barrier. Peak serum concentrations are achieved at 1–1.7 hours and the plasma half-life is 1.3 hours. It achieves good penetration into lung tissue and bronchial secretions. It is excreted in the urine as unchanged drug and metabolites.

Uses
Reduction of sputum viscosity

Contraindications
Active peptic ulceration

Administration
Orally: 750 mg 8–12 hourly

Adverse effects
Anaphylactic reactions
Skin rashes/allergy
Gastrointestinal bleeding

Renal replacement therapy
No dose adjustment is required

CASPOFUNGIN (Cancidas)

Caspofungin covers a wider range of *Candida* species causing invasive candidiasis than fluconazole and is active against *Aspergillus* species. It has a better side-effect profile than amphotericin. In mild liver failure, AUC is increased by 20% and moderate liver failure by 75%, hence the dose reduction in moderate liver failure. Side-effects are typically mild and rarely lead to discontinuation.

Uses
Invasive candidiasis
Invasive aspergillosis

Contraindications
Breastfeeding

Administration
- IV: Load with 70 mg on day 1, followed by 50 mg daily thereafter typically for at least 9 days
  If > 80 kg, continue with maintenance dose of 70 mg daily
  Reconstitute with 10 ml WFI. Add the reconstituted solution to a 100 ml or 250 ml bag of sodium chloride 0.9% or Hartmann's solution, given over 1 hour
  Available in vials containing 50 mg and 70 mg powder. Store vials in fridge at 2–8°C

How not to use caspofungin
Do not use diluents containing glucose

Adverse effects
Thrombophlebitis
Fever
Headache
Tachycardia
Anaemia
Decreased platelet count
Elevated LFT
Hypokalaemia
Hypomagnesaemia

Cautions
Co-administration with the inducers efavirenz, nevirapine, rifampicin, dexamethasone, phenytoin or carbamazepine may result in a decrease in caspofungin AUC, so increase in the daily dose of caspofungin to 70 mg. Ciclosporin increases the AUC of caspofungin by approximately 35%. Caspofungin lowers trough concentrations of tacrolimus by 26%

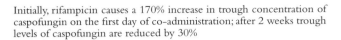

Initially, rifampicin causes a 170% increase in trough concentration of caspofungin on the first day of co-administration; after 2 weeks trough levels of caspofungin are reduced by 30%

Organ failure
Renal: No dose adjustment necessary
Hepatic: Mild (Child–Pugh score 5–6): no dose adjustment
Moderate (Child–Pugh score 7–9): 70 mg loading followed by 35 mg daily
Severe (Child–Pugh score >9): no data

Organ replacement therapy
Not removed by dialysis

CEFOTAXIME

C

A third-generation cephalosporin with enhanced activity against Gram −ve species in comparison with second-generation cephalosporins. It is not active against *Pseudomonas aeruginosa*, enterococci or *Bacteroides* spp. Use is increasingly being compromised by the emergence of Gram −ve strains expressing extended spectrum beta-lactamases (ESBLs) and chromosomal beta-lactamase producers.

Uses
Surgical prophylaxis, although first- and second-generation cephalosporins are usually preferred
Acute epiglottitis due to *Haemophilus influenzae*
Empiric therapy of meningitis
Intra-abdominal infections including peritonitis
Community-acquired and nosocomial pneumonia
Urinary tract infections
Sepsis of unknown origin

Contraindications
Hypersensitivity to cephalosporins
Serious penicillin hypersensitivity (10% cross-sensitivity)
Porphyria

Administration
- IV: 1 g 12 hourly, increased in life-threatening infections (e.g. meningitis) to 3 g 6 hourly

  Reconstitute with 10 ml WFI, given over 3–5 min

Infection	Dose (g)	Interval (h)
Mild–moderate	1	12
Moderate–serious	2	8
Life-threatening	3	6

Adverse effects
Hypersensitivity
Transient ↑ LFTs
Clostridium difficile-associated diarrhoea

C

Cautions
Concurrent use of nephrotoxic drugs (aminoglycosides, loop diuretics)
Severe renal impairment (halve dose)
False +ve urinary glucose (if tested for reducing substances)
False +ve Coombs' test

Organ failure
Renal: In severe renal impairment (<10 ml/min): 1 g every 8–12 hours

Renal replacement therapy
No further dose modification is required during renal replacement therapy

CEFTAZIDIME

A third–generation cephalosporin whose activity against Gram +ve organisms, most notably *S. aureus*, is diminished in comparison with second-generation cephalosporins, while action against Gram −ve organisms, including *Pseudomonas aeruginosa*, is enhanced. Ceftazidime is not active against enterococci, MRSA or *Bacteroides* spp.

Uses
Acute epiglottitis due to *Haemophilus influenzae*
Meningitis due to *Pseudomonas aeruginosa*
Intra–abdominal infections including peritonitis
Nosocomial pneumonia
Urinary tract infections
Severe sepsis of unknown origin
Febrile neutropenia

Contraindications
Hypersensitivity to cephalosporins
Serious penicillin hypersensitivity (10% cross–sensitivity)
Porphyria

Administration
• IV: 2 g 8 hourly

Reconstitute with 10 ml WFI, given over 3–5 min

Infection	Dose (g)	Interval (h)
Mild–moderate	0.5–1	12
Moderate–serious	1	8
Life-threatening	2	8

In renal impairment:

CC (ml/min)	Dose (g)	Interval (h)
31–50	1–2	12
16–30	1–2	24
6–15	0.5–1	24
<5	0.5–1	48

Adverse effects
Hypersensitivity
Transient ↑ LFTs
Clostridium difficile–associated diarrhoea

Cautions
Renal impairment (reduce dose)
Concurrent use of nephrotoxic drugs (aminoglycosides, loop diuretics)
False +ve urinary glucose (if tested for reducing substances)
False −ve Coombs' test

Renal replacement therapy
CVVH dependent on clearance rate as described in Short Notes Renal Replacement Therapy (p. 300–303) and CC table given previously. PD dialysed 500 mg–1 g every 24 hours. HD dialysed 500 mg–1 g every 24–48 hours

CEFTRIAXONE

A third-generation cephalosporin which is similar in many respects to cefotaxime, with enhanced activity against Gram −ve species in comparison to second generation cephalosporins. Ceftriaxone is not active against enterococci, MRSA, *Pseudomonas aeruginosa* or *Bacteroides* spp. Ceftriaxone has a prolonged serum half-life allowing for once-daily dosing. However, twice daily dosing is normally recommended for severe infections including meningitis.

Uses
Empiric therapy for meningitis
Intra-abdominal infections including peritonitis
Community-acquired or nosocomial pneumonia
Surgical prophylaxis, although first- and second-generation cephalosporins are usually preferred
Clearance of throat carriage in meningococcal disease

Contraindications
Hypersensitivity to cephalosporins
Serious penicillin hypersensitivity (10% cross-sensitivity)
Porphyria

Administration
• IV: 2 g once daily, increased to 2 g 12 hourly in severe infections
  Reconstitute 2-g vial with 40 ml of glucose 5% or sodium chloride 0.9% given over at least 30 min

In renal impairment:

CC (ml/min)	Dose (g)	Interval (h)
<10	2	24

How not to use ceftriaxone
Not to be dissolved in infusion fluids containing calcium (Hartmann's)

Adverse effects
Hypersensitivity
Transient ↑ liver enzymes
Clostridium difficile-associated diarrhoea

Renal replacement therapy
No dose reduction needed

CEFUROXIME

A second-generation cephalosporin widely used in combination with metronidazole in the postoperative period following most abdominal procedures. Has greater activity against *Staphylococcus aureus* (including penicillinase–producing strains) compared with the third-generation cephalosporins, but not active against MRSA, enterococcus, *Pseudomonas aeruginosa* or *Bacteroides* spp. It also has poor activity against penicillin–resistant strains of *Streptococcus pneumoniae*.

Uses
Surgical prophylaxis
Acute epiglottitis due to *Haemophilus influenzae*
Intra–abdominal infections including peritonitis
Community-acquired and nosocomial pneumonia
Urinary tract infections
Patients admitted from the community with sepsis of unknown origin
Soft tissue infections

Contraindications
Hypersensitivity to cephalosporins
Serious penicillin hypersensitivity (10% cross–sensitivity)
Meningitis (high relapse rate)
Porphyria

Administration
• IV: 0.75–1.5 g 6–8 hourly

Reconstitute with 20 ml WFI, given over 3–5 min

In renal impairment:

CC (ml/min)	Dose (g)	Interval (h)
20–50	0.75–1.5	8
10–20	0.75–1.5	8–12
<10	0.75–1.5	12–24

Adverse effects
Hypersensitivity
Transient ↑ LFTs
Clostridium difficile–associated diarrhoea

Cautions
Hypersensitivity to penicillins
Renal impairment

Renal replacement therapy
CVVH dialysed dependent on clearance rate as described in Short Notes Renal Replacement Therapy (p. 300–303) and CC table given previously. For PD and HD dose as in CC <10 ml/min, i.e. 750 mg to 1.5 g IV every 12–24 hours

CHLORDIAZEPOXIDE

Chlordiazepoxide is a benzodiazepine used to attenuate alcohol withdrawal symptoms, but also has a dependence potential. The risk of dependence is minimised by limiting the duration of treatment and reducing the dose gradually over 7–14 days. It is available as 5-mg and 10-mg capsules or tablets.

Uses
Alcohol withdrawal
Restlessness and agitation

Contraindications
Alcohol-dependent patients who continue to drink
Obstructive sleep apnoea
Severe hepatic impairment

Administration
• Alcohol withdrawal

Orally:

	Dose (mg) at:			
Day	08:00 h	12:00 h	18:00 h	22:00 h
1	30	30	30	30
2	25	25	25	25
3	20	20	20	20
4	10	10	10	10
5	5	5	5	5
6	–	5	5	5
7	–	–	5	5
8	–	–	–	5

• Restlessness and agitation

Orally: 10–30 mg 3 times daily

How not to use chlordiazepoxide
Prolonged use (risk of dependence)
Abrupt withdrawal

Adverse effects
Muscle weakness
Confusion
Ataxia
Hypotension

C

Cautions
Concurrent use of other CNS depressants will produce excessive sedation
Cardiac and respiratory disease – confusion may indicate hypoxia
Hepatic impairment – sedation can mask hepatic coma (avoid if severe)
Renal impairment – increased cerebral sensitivity

Organ failure
Hepatic: reduced clearance with accumulation. Can precipitate coma
Renal: increased cerebral sensitivity

CHLORDIAZEPOXIDE

CICLOSPORIN

Ciclosporin is a cyclic peptide molecule derived from a soil fungus. It is a potent nephrotoxin, producing interstitial renal fibrosis with tubular atrophy. Monitoring of ciclosporin blood level is essential.

Normal range: 100–300 µg/l

For renal transplants: lower end of range

For heart/lung/liver: upper end of range

For stem cell transplant: 200–600 µg/l – dependent upon donor, conditioning regimen and T-depletion of graft

Uses

Prevention of organ rejection after transplantation

Administration

- IV dose: 1–5 mg/kg/day

  To be diluted 1 in 20 to 1 in 100 with sodium chloride 0.9% or glucose 5%

  To be given over 2–6 h

  Infusion should be completed within 12 h if using PVC lines

  Switch to oral for long-term therapy

- Oral: 1.5 times IV dose given 12 hourly

  Monitor: Hepatic function

  Renal function

  Ciclosporin blood level (pre-dose sample)

How not to use ciclosporin

Must not be given as IV bolus

Do not infuse at ≥ 12 h if using PVC lines – leaching of phthalates from the PVC

Adverse effects

Enhanced renal sensitivity to insults

↑ Plasma urea and serum creatinine secondary to glomerulosclerosis

Hypertension – responds to conventional antihypertensives

Hepatocellular damage (↑ transaminases)

Hyperuricaemia

Gingival hypertrophy

Hirsutism

Tremors or seizures at high serum levels

Cautions

↑ Susceptibility to infections and lymphoma

↑ Nephrotoxic effects with concurrent use of other nephrotoxic drugs

CIPROFLOXACIN

Ciprofloxacin is a fluoroquinolone with bactericidal activity against *E. coli*, *Klebsiella* spp., *Proteus* spp., *Serratia* spp., *Salmonella* spp., *Campylobacter* spp., *Pseudomonas aeruginosa*, *Haemophilus influenzae*, *Neisseria* spp. and *Staphylococcus* spp. Many strains of MRSA in the UK are resistant and the use of ciprofloxacin may be associated with increased rates of MRSA and *C. difficile* colonisation. Activity against many other Gram +ve organisms is poor.

Uses
Respiratory tract infection − avoid if possibility of pneumococcal infection
Severe urinary tract infection
Intra-abdominal infections
Meningitis prophylaxis (unlicensed)
Severely ill patients with gastroenteritis
Suspected enteric fever
Sepsis of unknown origin

Administration
• For infection

    IV infusion: 200–400 mg 12 hourly, given over 30–60 min
    400 mg 8 hourly dosing may be required for *P. aeruginosa* and other less susceptible Gram −ve organisms
    Available in 100 ml bottle containing 200 mg ciprofloxacin in sodium chloride 0.9% and 200 ml bottle containing 400 mg ciprofloxacin in sodium chloride 0.9%. Contains Na^+ 15.4 mmol/100 ml bottle
    Also available in 100-ml bag containing 200 mg ciprofloxacin in glucose 5% and 200 ml bottle containing 400 mg ciprofloxacin in glucose 5%
    Oral: 500–750 mg 12 hourly

In renal impairment:

CC (ml/min)	Dose (% of normal dose)
20–50	100
10–20	50–100
<10	50 (100% if necessary for short periods)

• Meningitis prophylaxis

    Oral: 500 mg as a single dose or 12 hourly for 2 days
    Child 5–12 years: 250 mg orally, as a single dose

How not to use ciprofloxacin
Do not put in fridge (crystal formation)
Do not use as sole agent where pneumococcal infection likely

C

Adverse effects
Transient increases in bilirubin, liver enzymes and creatinine
Tendon damage and rupture, especially in the elderly and those taking
corticosteroids (may occur within 48 hours)

Cautions
Concurrent administration with theophylline (increased plasma level
of theophylline)
Concurrent administration with ciclosporin (transient increase in
serum creatinine)
Epilepsy (increased risk of fits)
Concurrent administration of corticosteroids (risk of tendon damage
and rupture)

Organ failure
Renal: reduce dose

Renal replacement therapy
No further dose modification is required during renal replacement
therapy

CLARITHROMYCIN

Clarithromycin is an erythromycin derivative with slightly greater activity, a longer half-life and higher tissue penetration than erythromycin. Adverse effects are thought to be less common than with erythromycin. Resistance rates in Gram +ve organisms limit its use for severe soft tissue infections.

Uses
Community-acquired pneumonia
Infective exacerbations of COPD
Pharyngeal and sinus infections
Soft tissue infections
Helicobacter pylori eradication as part of combination therapy with a proton pump inhibitor plus amoxicillin or metronidazole

Administration
- Orally: 250–500 mg 12 hourly
- IV: 500 mg 12 hourly

  Reconstitute in 10 ml WFI. Then make up to 250 ml with glucose 5% or sodium chloride 0.9% and give over 60 min

How not to use clarithromycin
Should not be given as IV bolus or IM injection

Adverse effects
Gastrointestinal intolerance
↑ LFTs (usually reversible)

Organ failure
Renal: no dose reduction necessary in renal failure

CLOMETHIAZOLE

Clomethiazole is available as capsules (192 mg) and syrup (250 mg/5 ml), but no longer available as a 0.8% solution for IV use. One capsule is equivalent to 5 ml syrup. The capsule contains 192 mg clomethiazole (base) while the syrup contains 250 mg clomethiazole edisilate per 5 ml. The difference in weight is due to the inactive edisilate group.

Uses
Alcohol withdrawal
Restlessness and agitation

Contraindications
Alcohol-dependent patients who continue to drink

Administration
1 capsule = 5 ml syrup

• Alcohol withdrawal

Oral: Day 1, 9–12 capsules in 3–4 divided doses
Day 2, 6–8 capsules in 3–4 divided doses
Day 3, 4–6 capsules in 3–4 divided doses
Then gradually reduce over days 4–6
Do not treat for >9 days

• Restlessness and agitation

Oral: 1 capsule 3 times daily

How not to use clomethiazole
Prolonged use (risk of dependence)
Abrupt withdrawal

Adverse effects
Increased nasopharyngeal and bronchial secretions
Conjunctival irritation
Headache

Cautions
Concurrent use of other CNS depressants will produce excessive sedation
Cardiac and respiratory disease – confusion may indicate hypoxia
Hepatic impairment – sedation can mask hepatic coma
Renal impairment

Organ failure
Hepatic: reduced clearance with accumulation. Can precipitate coma
Renal: increase cerebral sensitivity

CLONIDINE

Clonidine is an α_2-adrenoceptor agonist which may have a protective effect on cardiovascular morbidity and mortality in the critically ill patient. The mechanism of the protective effect is likely to be manifold. α_2-adrenoceptor agonists attenuate haemodynamic instability, inhibit central sympathetic discharge, reduce peripheral norepinephrine release and dilate post-stenotic coronary vessels. Its use as an antihypertensive agent has since been superseded by other drugs. It has a useful sedative property, which is synergistic with opioids and other sedative agents. It is a useful short-term adjuvant to sedation especially following extubation where there is a high sympathetic drive and in the agitated patient. Its usage should not usually exceed 3 days, as withdrawal can lead to rebound hypertension and agitation.

Uses
Short-term adjunct to sedation (unlicensed)

Contraindications
Hypotension
Porphyria

Administration
- Orally: 50 µg 8 hourly, may be increased gradually to 400 µg 8 hourly
- IV bolus: 50 µg 8 hourly, given slowly over 10–15 min, may be increased gradually to 250 µg 8 hourly
- IV infusion: 30–100 µg/h

  Available as 150 µg clonidine hydrochloride in 1 ml ampoule (Catapres)
  750 µg (5 ampoules) made up to 50 ml with glucose 5% or sodium chloride 0.9% (15 µg/ml)

How not to use clonidine
Sudden withdrawal if used for longer than 3 days

Adverse effects
Bradycardia
Hypotension
Fluid retention
Dry mouth
Sedation
Depression
Constipation

C

Cautions

Avoid prolonged use and sudden withdrawal (rebound hypertension)
Peripheral vascular disease (concomitant use with beta blockers may worsen condition)
Second-degree heart block (may progress to complete heart block)
Avoid concomitant use with:

Beta-blockers (bradycardia)
Tricyclics (counteract effect)
NSAIDs (sodium and water retention)
Digoxin (bradycardia)
Haloperidol (prolongation of QT interval)

Organ failure

Renal: no dose reduction necessary in renal failure, though plasma levels are higher in severe renal dysfunction

CLONIDINE

CLOPIDOGREL

In addition to standard therapy (aspirin, LMWH, β-blocker and nitrate), clopidogrel reduces the risk of MI, stroke and cardiovascular death in patients with unstable angina and non–ST-elevation MI (The CURE investigators. *N Engl J Med* 2001; **345**: 494–502). NICE and the European Society of Cardiology both endorse the use of clopidogrel in combination with aspirin in non–ST-elevation acute coronary syndrome patients. Clopidogrel is also used with aspirin in STEMI and after angioplasty for up to 12 months.

Clopidogrel is a prodrug that is metabolised to an active form, primarily via cytochrome P450 2C19. PPIs inhibit this enzyme to varying degrees, and mechanistic studies show that combined use of clopidogrel with omeprazole or lansoprazole leads to a reduction in activity of clopidogrel as measured by platelet aggregation and associated biomarkers. Avoid omeprazole and esomeprazole in combination with clopidogrel. Pantoprazole is the most appropriate PPI to use in combination. Lansoprazole and rabeprazole are alternatives, but pharmacokinetic data is lacking. There is insufficient data to determine the significance of these interactions. The balance of risks and benefits should guide decision making.

Uses
Acute coronary syndrome, prevention of atherothrombotic events in peripheral arterial disease or after myocardial infarction or ischaemic stroke, prevention of atherothrombotic and thromboembolic events in patients with atrial fibrillation

Contraindications
Warfarin
Severe liver impairment
Active bleeding
Breast feeding

Administration
Unstable angina and non–ST-elevation MI: single 300 mg loading dose (or 600 mg is an unlicensed loading dose that may produce a greater and quicker inhibition of platelet aggregation), followed by 75 mg daily (with aspirin 75 mg/day) for up to 12 months. AF 75 mg daily (with aspirin), prevention of artherothrombotic events 75 mg daily

Monitor:
> FBC
> Clotting screen
> Discontinue 7 days prior to surgery

How not to use clopidogrel
Omit clopidogrel if patient likely to go for CABG within 5 days
Not recommended under 18 years of age
Pregnancy

Adverse effects
Bleeding (can protect with ranitidine)
Abnormal LFTs and raised serum creatinine
Haematological disorders including pancytopenia

Cautions
Avoid for 7 days after ischaemic stroke
Increase risk of bleeding with the concurrent use of:
aspirin (although recommended for up to 12 months in CURE study)
NSAIDs
heparin
thrombolytics
glycoprotein IIb/IIIa inhibitors

Avoid concomitant use of PPIs, fluoxetine, fluconazole, ciprofloxacin and carbamazepine (clopidogrel may be less effective)

Organ failure
Hepatic: avoid in severe liver impairment

C

CLOPIDOGREL

CO-AMOXICLAV

Amoxicillin + clavulanic acid (β-lactamase inhibitor). The β-lactamase inhibitory action of clavulinic acid extends the spectrum of antibacterial activity of amoxicillin.

Uses
Respiratory tract infections
Genito-urinary tract infections
Intra-abdominal sepsis
Surgical prophylaxis

Contraindications
Penicillin hypersensitivity

Administration
- IV: 1.2 g 8 hourly (6 hourly in severe infections)
  Reconstitute with 20 ml WFI, given IV over 3–5 min

In renal impairment:

Initial dose of 1.2 g, then:

CC (ml/min)	Dose (g)	Interval (h)
10–20	1.2	12
<10	0.6–1.2	12

How not to use co-amoxiclav
Do not mix with aminoglycoside in same syringe (will inactivate aminoglycoside)

Adverse effects
Hypersensitivity
Cholestatic jaundice (usually self-limiting, up to 2–6 weeks after treatment stops)
Bleeding and prothrombin time may be prolonged

Organ failure
Renal: reduce dose

Renal replacement therapy
CVVH dialysed dependent on clearance rate as described in Short Notes Renal Replacement Therapy (p. 300–303) and CC table given previously; oral as for normal renal function. HD and PD dialysed dose as in CC <10 ml/min, i.e. IV: 1.2 g *stat* followed by 600 mg–1.2 g every 12 hours; oral 375–625 mg 8 hourly. Pharmacokinetics of the amoxicillin and clauvulanate are closely matched, probably cleared at similar rates

CODEINE PHOSPHATE

C

Codeine has a low affinity for the $\mu(OP_3)$ and $k(OP_2)$ opioid receptors.
It is relatively more effective when given orally than parenterally. It is
useful as an antitussive and for the treatment of diarrhoea. Sideeffects
are uncommon and respiratory depression is seldom a problem. This
explains its traditional use to provide analgesia for head-injured and
neurosurgical patients. Doses >60 mg do not improve analgesic activity
but may increase side-effects. 10% undergoes demethylation to morphine – this possibly contributing to the analgesic effect.

Uses
Mild to moderate pain
Diarrhoea and excessive ileostomy output
Antitussive

Contraindications
Airway obstruction

Administration
- Orally: 30–60 mg 4–6 hourly
- IM: 30–60 mg 4–6 hourly

How not to use codeine phosphate
Not for IV use

Adverse effects
Drowsiness
Constipation
Nausea and vomiting
Respiratory depression

Cautions
Enhanced sedative and respiratory depression from interaction with:

- benzodiazepines
- antidepressants
- anti-psychotics

MAOI (hypertension, hyperpyrexia, convulsions and coma)
Head injury and neurosurgical patients (may exacerbate $\uparrow$ ICP as a
result of $\uparrow$ $PaCO_2$)
May cause renal failure

Organ failure
CNS: sedative effects increased
Hepatic: can precipitate coma
Renal: increase cerebral sensitivity

Renal replacement therapy
No further dose modification is required during renal replacement
therapy

CO-TRIMOXAZOLE

Sulphamethoxazole and trimethoprim are used in combination because of their synergistic activity. Increasing resistance to sulphonamides and the high incidence of sulphonamide–related side–effects have diminished the value of co-trimoxazole. Trimethoprim alone is now preferred for urinary tract infections and exacerbations of chronic bronchitis. However, high–dose co-trimoxazole is the preferred treatment for *Pneumocystis carinii* pneumonia (PCP). It has certain theoretical advantages over pentamidine: pentamidine accumulates slowly in the lung parenchyma and improvement may occur more slowly; co-trimoxazole has a broad spectrum of activity and may treat any bacterial co–pathogens. Pneumonia caused by *Pneumocystis carinii* (now renamed *Pneumocystis jirovecii*) occurs in immunosuppressed patients; it is a common cause of pneumonia in AIDS. High–dose co-trimoxazole with corticosteroid therapy is the treatment of choice for moderate to severe infections. Co-trimoxazole prophylaxis should be considered for severely immunocompromised patients.

Uses
Pneumocystis carinii pneumonia

Contraindications
Pregnancy
Severe renal/hepatic failure
Blood disorders
Porphyria

Administration
- Can infuse undiluted solution via central line (unlicensed)
- *Pneumocystis carinii* pneumonia

  60 mg/kg 12 hourly IV for 14 days followed orally for a further 7 days. Some units reduce the dose from day 3 to 45 mg/kg 12 hourly as this appears to reduce side effects but maintain efficacy. IV infusion: dilute every 1 ml (96 mg) in 25 ml glucose 5% or sodium chloride 0.9%, given over 1.5–2 h. If fluid restriction necessary, dilute in half the amount of glucose 5%

  Adjuvant corticosteroid has been shown to improve survival. The steroid should be started at the same time as the co-trimoxazole and should be withdrawn before the antibiotic treatment is complete. Oral prednisolone 50–80 mg daily or IV hydrocortisone 100 mg 6 hourly or IV dexamethasone 8 mg 6 hourly or IV methylprednisolone 1 g for 5 days, then dose reduced to complete 21 days of treatment

- PCP prophylaxis

  Oral: 960 mg daily or 960 mg on alternate days (3 times a week) or 480 mg daily to improve tolerance

C

• In renal impairment

CC 15–30 ml/min: reduce dose to 50% after day 3 for PCP treatment CC <15 ml/min: reduce dose to 50%; should only be given with renal replacement therapy

Note: treatment should be stopped if rashes or serious blood disorders develop. A fall in white cell count should be treated with folic/folinic acid and a dose reduction to 75%

How not to use co-trimoxazole
Concurrent use of co-trimoxazole and pentamidine is not of benefit and may increase the incidence of serious side-effects

Adverse effects
Nausea, vomiting and diarrhoea (including pseudomembranous colitis)
Rashes (including Stevens–Johnson syndrome)
Blood disorders (includes leucopenia, thrombocytopenia, anaemia)
Fluid overload (due to large volumes required)

Cautions
Elderly
Renal impairment (rashes and blood disorders increase, may cause further deterioration in renal function)

Renal replacement therapy
CVVH dialysed, normal dose for the first three days then dependent on clearance rate as described in Short Notes Renal Replacement Therapy and renal impairment information given previously (p. 300–303). PD not dialysed, dose as for HD

CO-TRIMOXAZOLE

C

CYCLIZINE

Antihistamine with antimuscarinic effects.

Uses
Nausea and vomiting

Administration
• IM/IV: 50 mg 8 hourly

Adverse effects
Anticholinergic: drowsiness, dryness of mouth, blurred vision, tachycardia

Cautions
Sedative effect enhanced by concurrent use of other CNS depressants

Organ failure
CNS: sedative effects enhanced

DALTEPARIN (Fragmin)

D

A low molecular weight heparin (LMWH) with greater anti-Factor Xa activity than anti-IIa (antithrombin) activity, which theoretically makes it more effective at preventing thrombin formation than standard (unfractionated) heparin with an equal anti-Factor Xa and anti-IIa ratio.

After SC injection, LMWHs are better absorbed than unfractionated heparin, and bind less to proteins in plasma and in the endothelial wall. As a result they have around 90% bioavailability compared with 10–30% with unfractionated heparin. After SC injection, the plasma half-life of LMWHs is around 4 hours, enabling a single dose to provide effective anti-coagulant activity for up to 24 hours in the treatment of venous thromboembolism, peri- and postoperative surgical thomboprophylaxis, and the prevention of clotting in the extracorporeal circulation during haemodialysis or haemofiltration.

The incidence of bleeding is similar between LMWHs and unfractionated heparin. The incidence of immune-mediated thrombocytopenia is about 2–3% of patients treated with unfractionated heparin, typically developing after 5–10 days' treatment. In clinical trials with dalteparin, thrombocytopenia occurred in up to 1% of patients receiving treatment for unstable angina, undergoing abdominal surgery or hip replacement surgery.

LMWHs are preferred over unfractionated heparin because they are as effective, simplify treatment (once-daily dosing, no IV cannulation), have a lower risk of heparin-induced thrombocytopenia and monitoring is not required.

Uses
Prophylaxis of DVT
Treatment of DVT and pulmonary embolism or both
Unstable angina
Prevention of clotting in extracorporeal circuits

Contraindications
Generalised bleeding tendencies
Acute GI ulcer
Cerebral haemorrhage
Subacute endocarditis
Heparin-induced immune thrombocytopenia
Injuries to and operations on the CNS, eyes and ears
Known haemorrhagic diathesis
Hypersensitivity to dalteparin or other LMWHs and/or heparins

D

Administration

- Peri- and post-operative surgical prophylaxis – moderate risk 2,500 units only daily SC
- Peri- and post-operative surgical prophylaxis – high risk 5000 units once daily SC >100 kg 5,000 units twice daily SC, >150 kg 7,500 units twice daily SC (unlicensed dose)
- Prophylaxis of DVT in medical patients 5000 units once daily SC >100 kg 5,000 units twice daily SC, >150 kg 7,500 units twice daily SC (unlicensed dose)

Consider dose reduction to 2,500 units SC daily if weight <45 kg, frail elderly or CC <30 ml/min. Lumbar puncture, epidural insertion/ removal, etc. avoid prophylactic dose dalteparin 12 hours before and 4 hours post procedure (12 hours if traumatic)

- Treatment of DVT and pulmonary embolus or both

  Start dalteparin with oral warfarin (as soon as possible) until INR in therapeutic range
  200 units/kg once daily SC up to maximum daily dose of 18,000 units or 100 units/kg twice daily if increased risk of haemorrhage

Actual body weight (kg)	Dose (200 units/kg)
<46	7,500 once daily SC
46–56	10,000 once daily SC
57–68	12,500 once daily SC
69–82	15,000 once daily SC
83–99	18,000 once daily SC
100–110	10,000 twice daily SC
>110	an increased (unlicensed) dose may be warranted (given in two divided doses), with anti-Xa monitoring

- Unstable angina

  Acute phase: 120 units/kg 12 hourly SC
  Maximum dose: 10,000 units twice daily
  Concomitant treatment with low-dose aspirin
  Recommended treatment period up to 8 days

  - Extended phase: men <70 kg, 5,000 units once daily SC, >70 kg 7,500 units once daily SC
  - Women <80 kg 5,000 units once daily SC, >80 kg 7,500 units once daily SC

  Treatment should not be given for more than 45 days
  Monitor: platelets
  APTT monitoring is not usually required
  In overdose, 100 units dalteparin is inhibited by 1 mg protamine

D

Adverse effects

Subcutaneous haematoma at injection site

Bleeding at high doses, e.g., anti–Factor Xa levels greater than 1.5 iu/ml; however, at recommended doses bleeding rarely occurs

Transient increase in liver enzymes (ALT) but no clinical significance has been demonstrated

Rarely thrombocytopenia

Rarely hypoaldosteronism resulting in increased plasma potassium, particularly in chronic renal failure, diabetes mellitus or pre-existing metabolic acidosis

Organ failure

Renal: ideally avoid for treatment doses where CC <30 ml/min; replace with unfractionated heparin, as accumulation will occur, alternatively, use enoxaparin (p. 85) 1 mg/kg once daily.

If essential, dalteparin can be given in 2 divided doses (unlicensed dose):

CC 20–25 ml/min: 2/3 treatment dose

CC 25–30 ml/min: 3/4 treatment dose

CC <20 ml/min: 50% treatment dose

There is an increased risk of bleeding in renal failure and anti-Xa level monitoring is often necessary.

For thromboprophylactic doses, it appears safe to use dalteparin 2500 units SC once daily.

Renal replacement therapy

Treatment doses of LMWHs are generally avoided in renal replacement therapy, since anti-Xa monitoring is required to use safely. The use of unfractionated heparin is preferred

DALTEPARIN (Fragmin)

D

DANAPAROID (Orgaran)

Danaparoid preferentially acts on antifactor-Xa rather than anti-thrombin and hence therapy is monitored via anti-Xa levels. For full anticoagulation anti-Xa target 0.5–0.8 iu/ml; levels >2 iu/ml may lead to serious bleeding complications. It is licensed for prophylaxis and treatment of DVT and pulmonary embolism. It is an option in ICU patients with heparin-induced thrombocytopenia (HIT) who need anticoagulation and haemofiltration (unlicensed). Cross-reactivity with HIT IgG antibody may occur in less than 10% of cases and cannot be predicted by *in vitro* testing prior to onset of therapy.

There is no antidote to its effects, although its action may be partially reversed by protamine. The anti-Xa half-life is 25 hours. Steady-state levels occur after 5 days of therapy in constant conditions. Danaparoid is 50% renally excereted so dose reductions may be required in renal failure and renal replacement therapy.

Uses
Anticoagulation for patients with HIT

Contraindications
Haemophilia and other haemorrhagic disorders
Thrombocytopenia (except HIT)
Recent cerebral haemorrhage
Severe hypertension
Active peptic ulcer (unless this is the reason for operation)
Diabetic retinopathy
Acute bacterial endocarditis
Spinal or epidural anaesthesia with treatment doses of danaparoid

Administration
Danaparoid available in 2 strengths:
    0.6 ml ampoule containing 750 units
    1 ml ampoule containing 1250 units

• Prophylaxis of DVT and PE

    SC: 750 units SC 12 hourly

• Treatment of DVT and PE

    IV: loading dose (weight dependent) followed by continuous IV infusion

IV loading dose (undiluted) over 15–30 seconds:

Weight (kg)	Loading dose (units)	Volume of danaparoid 750 units/0.6 ml (ml)
<55 kg	1,250 units	1 ml
55–90 kg	2,500 units	2 ml
>90 kg	3,750 units	3 ml

DANAPAROID (Orgaran)

D

Followed by IV infusion:
Prepare infusion as follows:

1. Draw up 4 ml of the 750 units/0.6 ml danaparoid solution (5,000 units) into a 50-ml syringe
2. Dilute to 50-ml with either sodium chloride 0.9% or glucose 5%

This solution contains 5,000 units in 50 ml (100 units in 1 ml)

Using a standard strength solution of 100 units in 1 ml

Dose	Infusion rate (ml/hour)	Duration
400 units/h	4	2 hours
300 units/h	3	2 hours
200 units/h	2	5 days (is there a time limit?)

- HIT in haemofiltration

IV loading dose (as previously), then 100 units/h continuous IV infusion, increasing to 200 units/h only if the filter clots or if levels are low and full anticoagulation is required. Monitor anti-Xa levels regularly (e.g. daily)

The IV bolus and infusions can be given by peripheral or central vein

Monitoring of danaparoid
Plasma anti-Xa levels are used to monitor the effects of danaparoid. In general, they are not necessary but should be used if the patient has renal impairment, is on CVVH or is greater than 90 kg in weight

Anti-Xa levels have to be sent to specialist units for assay. Contact your haematology lab. for advice. Two samples must be collected in citrate bottles (green tube). Sample tubes must be full in order to obtain a viable result

	Expected levels
5 to 10 minutes after loading dose	0.5–0.7 units/ml
Adjustment phase of infusion	Not greater than 1 unit/ml
Maintenance infusion	0.5–0.8 units/ml
Patients on CVVH maintenance	0.5–1 units/ml

DANAPAROID (Orgaran)

D

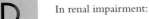

In renal impairment:

GFR ml/min

20–50	Dose as in normal renal function
10–20	Use with caution
<10	Use with caution. Reduce second and subsequent doses for thromboembolism prophylaxis

Adverse effects
Pain at injection site
Bruising
Bleeding
Hypersensitivity reactions (including rash)

Organ failure
Renal: reduce dose

Renal replacement therapy
For haemofiltration, see under administration

DANTROLENE

D

Dantrolene is thought to work in MH by interfering with the release of calcium from sarcoplasmic reticulum to the myoplasm. The average dose required to reverse the manifestations of MH is 2.5 mg/kg. If a relapse or recurrence occurs, dantrolene should be re-administered at the last effective dose. When used for the short-term treatment of MH there are usually no side-effects. Dantrolene has been used in the treatment of hyperthermia and rhabdomyolysis caused by theophylline overdose, consumption of 'Ecstasy' and 'Eve', and in the neuroleptic malignant syndrome and thyrotoxic storm. Neuroleptic malignant syndrome is characterised by hyperthermia, muscle rigidity, tachycardia, labile BP, sweating, autonomic dysfunction, urinary incontinence and fluctuating level of consciousness. It has been reported with haloperidol, fluphenazine, chlorpromazine, droperidol, thioridazine, metoclopramide, flupenthixol decanoate and tricyclic antidepressants.

Uses
MH (p. 261)
Neuroleptic malignant syndrome (unlicensed)
Thyrotoxic storm (unlicensed)
Hyperthermia and rhabdomyolysis associated with theophylline overdose, consumption of 'Ecstasy' and 'Eve' (unlicensed)

Contraindications
Hepatic impairment (worsens)

Administration
• IV: 1 mg/kg, repeated PRN up to 10 mg/kg

  Reconstitute each 20 mg vial with 60 ml WFI and shake well
  Each vial contains a mixture of 20 mg dantrolene sodium, 3 g mannitol and sodium hydroxide to yield a pH 9.5 when reconstituted with 60 ml WFI

Adverse effects
Rash
Diarrhoea
Muscle weakness
Hepatotoxicity

Cautions
Concurrent use of diltiazem (arrhythmias)
Concurrent use of calcium channel blockers (hypotension, myocardial depression and hyperkalaemia reported with verapamil)

DANTROLENE

DESMOPRESSIN (DDAVP)

Pituitary diabetes insipidus (DI) results from a deficiency of antidiuretic hormone (ADH) secretion. Desmopressin is an analogue of ADH. Treatment may be required for a limited period only in DI following head trauma or pituitary surgery. It is also used in the differential diagnosis of DI. Restoration of the ability to concentrate urine after water deprivation confirms a diagnosis of pituitary DI. Failure to respond occurs in nephrogenic DI.

Uses
Pituitary DI – diagnosis and treatment

Administration
- Diagnosis
  Intranasally: 20 µg
  SC/IM: 2 µg

- Treatment

  Intranasally: 5–20 µg once or twice daily
  SC/IM/IV: 1–4 µg daily
  Monitor fluid intake
  Patient should be weighed daily
  Orally: 100–200 µg three times per day (range 50 µg twice daily up to 400 µg three times per day)

Adverse effects
Fluid retention
Hyponatraemia
Headache
Nausea and vomiting

Cautions
Renal impairment
Cardiac disease
Hypertension
Cystic fibrosis (risk of hypernatraemia)

DEXAMETHASONE

Dexamethasone has very high glucocorticoid activity and insignificant mineralocorticoid activity, making it particularly suitable for conditions where water retention would be a disadvantage. Adjuvant corticosteroid has been shown to improve survival in *Pneumocystis carinii* pneumonia. It is also a useful anti-emetic when others are contraindicated or ineffective. Its effects are additive to 5-HT$_3$ antagonists.

Uses
Cerebral oedema
Laryngeal oedema
Adjunct in *Pneumocystis carinii* pneumonia (see co-trimoxazole and pentamidine)
Bacterial meningitis, particularly where pneumococcal suspected
Nausea and vomiting

Contraindications
Systemic infection (unless specific anti-microbial therapy given)

Administration
* Cerebral oedema

    IV bolus: 8 mg initially, then 4 mg 6 hourly as required for 2–10 days

* *Pneumocystis carinii* pneumonia

    IV bolus: 8 mg 6 hourly 5 days, then dose reduced to complete 21 days of treatment
    The steroid should be started at the same time as the co-trimoxazole or pentamidine and should be withdrawn before the antibiotic treatment is complete

* nausea and vomiting 4–8 mg po/iv 12 hourly. Give the 2nd dose early afternoon to reduce insomnia.

How not to use dexamethasone
Do not stop abruptly after prolonged use (adrenocortical insufficiency)

Adverse effects
Perineal irritation may follow IV administration of the phosphate ester
Prolonged use may also lead to the following problems:

* increased susceptibility to infections
* impaired wound healing
* peptic ulceration
* muscle weakness (proximal myopathy)

- osteoporosis
- hyperglycaemia
- agitation
- insomnia

Cautions
Diabetes mellitus
Concurrent use of NSAID (increased risk of GI bleeding)

DEXMEDETOMIDINE

D

This sedative provides a unique type of sedation, which differs from other agents in terms of the ability to rouse during sedation. Its mechanism of action is similar to clonidine, i.e. it is a selective alpha-2 receptor agonist. The PRODEX and MIDEX trials (*JAMA* 2012; **307**:1151–1160) compared dexmedetomidine to propofol and midazolam, respectively. It reported a shorter time for mechanical ventilation for dexmedetomidine compared to midazolam but not propofol; length of stay was similar in ICU and hospital. Dexmedetomidine patients experienced increased hypotension and bradycardia compared with midazolam, although patients were more interactive than with midazolam and propofol. Dexmedetomidine patients had a quicker time to extubation.

The key features of dexmedetomidine are a quick onset and offset of action (the half-life is 90 minutes), and it does not accumulate in renal dysfunction as it is liver metabolised and it generally does not course respiratory depression. There are a subset of patients who get inadequate sedation from this drug

While most of the trial data focuses on general sedation, there may be particular benefits of this drug in certain subgroups such as:

NIV, where sedation is deemed beneficial or necessary to tolerate, but where respiratory depression from standard sedatives is undesirable and may lead to unnecessary intubation

Weaning off mechanical ventilation: in the terminal phase of weaning off sedation as an alternative to propofol (where haemodynamic compromise is undesirable) and midazolam (with inherent risks of ICU delirium) as a bridge to analgesia only

In 'difficult to sedate' patients, as an alternative to clonidine if they do not respond well to it, or if there is a concern of haemodynamic compromise

Others have used dexmedetomidine for insomnia and delirium

Uses
Sedation of adult ICU patients requiring a sedation level not deeper than rousal in response to verbal stimulation [corresponding to Richmond Agitation–Sedation Scale (RASS) 0 to -3]

Contraindications
Advanced heart block (grade 2 or 3) unless paced
Uncontrolled hypotension
Acute cerebrovascular conditions
Hypersensitivity to dexmedetomidine or excipients

D

Administration
• Patients already intubated and sedated – initial infusion rate of 0.7 µg/kg/h, which may then be adjusted stepwise within the dose range 0.2–1.4 µg/kg/h in order to achieve the desired level of sedation, depending on the patient's response. Propofol or midazolam may be administered if needed until clinical effects are established

Avoid use a loading dose as it is associated with increased adverse reactions

Administer centrally or via a large peripheral line. Dilute in glucose 5%, sodium chloride 0.9% or Hartmann's to a final volume of 4 µg/ml; e.g. 2 ml of 100 µg/ml concentrate in 48 ml of diluent. However, in fluid restriction, concentrations up to 10.5 µg/ml have been used in trials (unlicensed), and 1000 µg in 50 ml in practice.

How not to use
Do not use a loading dose as this increases bradycardia and hypotension

Adverse effects
Hypotension incidence 25% (serious 1.7%), hypertension 15% and bradycardia 13% (serious 0.9%)
Myocardial ischaemia/infarction, tachycardia
Hyper-/hypoglycaemia
Nausea/vomiting, dry mouth
Withdrawal syndrome, hyperthermia

Renal replacement therapy
No dose adjustment is required

DIAZEPAM

D

Available formulated in either propylene glycol or a lipid emulsion (diazemuls), which causes minimal thrombophlebitis. Also available in a rectal solution (Stesolid) which takes up to 10 min to work.

Uses
Termination of epileptic fit

Contraindications
Airway obstruction

Administration
- IV: Diazemuls 5–10 mg over 2 min, repeated if necessary after 15 min, up to total 30 mg
- PR: Stesolid up to 20 mg

How not to use diazepam
IM injection – painful and unpredictable absorption

Adverse effects
Respiratory depression and apnoea
Drowsiness
Hypotension and bradycardia

Cautions
Airway obstruction with further neurological damage
Enhanced and prolonged sedative effect in the elderly
Additive effects with other CNS depressants

Organ failure
CNS: enhanced and prolonged sedative effect
Respiratory: ↑ respiratory depression
Hepatic: enhanced and prolonged sedative effect. Can precipitate coma
Renal: enhanced and prolonged sedative effect

Renal replacement therapy
No further dose modification is required during renal replacement therapy

DICLOFENAC

NSAID with analgesic, anti-inflammatory and antipyretic properties. It has an opioid-sparing effect. In the critically ill, the side-effects of NSAID are such that they have to be used with extreme caution – especially where there is a risk of stress ulceration, and renal impairment and bleeding diatheses are common. Ensure patient is adequately hydrated.

Uses
Pain, especially musculoskeletal
Antipyretic (unlicensed)

Contraindications
Uncontrolled asthma
Hypersensitivity to aspirin and other NSAID (cross-sensitivity)
Active peptic ulceration (bleeding)
Haemophilia and other clotting disorders (bleeding)
Renal and hepatic impairment (worsens)
Hypovolaemia
Anticoagulants including low-dose heparin (bleeding) with IV diclofenac

Administration
• Pain

    PO/NG: 50 mg 8 hourly
    PR: 100 mg suppository 18 hourly
    IV infusion: 75 mg diluted with 100–500 ml sodium chloride 0.9% or glucose 5%. For Voltarol: buffer the solution with sodium bicarbonate (0.5 ml 8.4% or 1 ml 4.2%)
    Give over 30–120 min
    Once prepared use immediately
    There is now a preparation of diclofenac called Dyloject which does not need diluting or buffering, and can be given as an IV bolus over 3–5 min
    Maximum daily dose: 150 mg

• Antipyretic

    IV bolus: 10 mg diluted with 20 ml sodium chloride 0.9%, given over 3 min

How not to use diclofenac
Do not give suppository in inflammatory bowel disease affecting anus, rectum and sigmoid colon (worsening of disease)

Adverse effects
Epigastric pain
Peptic ulcer
Rashes
Worsening of liver function tests

Prolonged bleeding time (platelet dysfunction)
Acute renal failure – in patients with:

- pre-existing renal and hepatic impairment
- hypovolaemia
- renal hypoperfusion
- sepsis

Cautions
Elderly
Hypovolaemia
Renal and hepatic impairment
Previous peptic ulceration

Organ failure
Hepatic: worsens
Renal: worsens

D

DICLOFENAC

DIGOXIN

A cardiac glycoside with both anti-arrhythmic and inotropic properties. Digoxin is useful for controlling the ventricular response in AF and atrial flutter.

Heart failure may also be improved. It is principally excreted unchanged by the kidney and will therefore accumulate in renal impairment.

Uses
SVT

Contraindications
Intermittent complete heart block
Second-degree AV block
WPW syndrome
Hypertrophic obstructive cardiomyopathy
Constrictive pericarditis

Administration
Digoxin: conversion factor from oral to IV = 0.67
i.e. 125 µg PO = 80 µg IV
- IV loading dose: 0.5–1.0 mg in 50 ml glucose 5% or sodium chloride 0.9%, given over 2 hours
- Maintenance dose: 62.5–250 µg daily (renal function is the most important determinant of maintenance dosage)

  CC 10–20 ml/min, i.e. 125–250 µg per day
  CC < 10 ml/min, i.e. 62.5 µg on alternate days or 62.5 µg daily

Monitor:

- ECG
- Serum digoxin level (p. 250)

How not to use digoxin
IM injections not recommended

Adverse effects
Anorexia, nausea, vomiting
Diarrhoea, abdominal pain
Visual disturbances, headache
Fatigue, drowsiness, confusion, delirium, hallucinations
Arrhythmias – all forms
Heart block

D

Cautions

Absorption from oral administration reduced by sucralfate and ion-exchange resins, colestyramine and colestipol

Hypokalaemia and hypomagnesaemia increase the sensitivity to digoxin, and the following drugs may predispose to toxicity:

- amphotericin
- β_2 sympathomimetics
- corticosteroids
- loop diuretics
- thiazides

Hypercalcaemia is inhibitory to the positive inotropic action of digoxin and potentiates the toxic effects
Plasma concentration of digoxin increased by:

- amiodarone
- diltiazem
- nicardipine
- propafenone
- quinidine
- verapamil

Digoxin toxicity (DC shock may cause fatal ventricular arrhythmia) – stop digoxin at least 24 h before cardioversion
β-Blockers and verapamil increase AV block and bradycardia
Suxamethonium predisposes to arrhythmias

Organ failure

Renal: toxicity – reduce dose, monitor levels

Renal replacement therapy

CVVH dependent on clearance rate as described in Short Notes Renal Replacement Therapy (pp. 300–303) and CC dosing information given previously and measured plasma levels. HD and PD not dialysed, dose as in CC <10 ml/min, i.e. 62.5 μg on alternate days or 62.5 μg daily; monitor levels

DIGOXIN

DOBUTAMINE

Dobutamine has predominant β_1 effects that increase heart rate and force of contraction. It also has mild β_2 and α_1 effects and decreases peripheral and pulmonary vascular resistance. Systolic BP may be increased because of the augmented cardiac output. Dobutamine has no specific effects on renal or splanchnic blood flow, but may increase renal blood flow due to an increase in cardiac output.

Uses
Low cardiac output states

Contraindications
Before adequate intravascular volume replacement
Idiopathic hypertrophic subaortic stenosis

Administration
• IV infusion: 1–25 µg/kg/min via a central vein

Titrate dose according to HR, BP, cardiac output, presence of ectopic beats and urine output
250 mg made up to 50 ml glucose 5% or sodium chloride 0.9% (5000 µg/ml)
Dosage chart (ml/h)

Weight (kg)	Dose (µg/kg/min)					
	2.5	5.0	7.5	10	15	20
50	1.5	3.0	4.5	6.0	9.0	12.0
60	1.8	3.6	5.4	7.2	10.8	14.5
70	2.1	4.2	6.3	8.4	12.75	16.8
80	2.4	4.8	7.2	9.6	14.4	19.2
90	2.7	5.4	8.1	10.8	16.2	21.6
100	3.0	6.0	9.0	12.0	18.0	24.0
110	3.3	6.6	9.9	13.2	19.8	26.4
120	3.6	7.2	10.8	14.4	21.6	28.8

D

How not to use dobutamine

In the absence of invasive cardiac monitoring
Inadequate correction of hypovolaemia before starting dobutamine
Do not connect to CVP lumen used for monitoring pressure (surge of drug during flushing of line)
Incompatible with alkaline solutions, e.g. sodium bicarbonate, furosemide, phenytoin and enoximone

Adverse effects

Tachycardia
Ectopic beats

Cautions

Acute myocardial ischaemia or MI
β–Blockers (may cause dobutamine to be less effective)

DOPAMINE

A naturally occurring catecholamine that acts directly on α, β_1 and dopaminergic receptors and indirectly by releasing noradrenaline.

- At low doses (0.5–2.5 µg/kg/min) it increases renal and mesenteric blood flow by stimulating dopamine receptors. The ↑ renal blood flow results in ↑ GFR and ↑ renal sodium excretion
- Doses between 2.5 and 10 µg/kg/min stimulate β_1 receptors causing ↑ myocardial contractility, stroke volume and cardiac output
- Doses >10 µg/kg/min stimulate α receptors causing ↑ SVR, ↓ renal blood flow and ↑ potential for arrhythmias

The distinction between dopamine's predominant dopaminergic and β effects at low doses and α effects at higher doses is not helpful in clinical practice due to marked inter-individual variation.

Uses
Septic shock
Low cardiac output

Contraindications
Attempt to increase urine output in patients inadequately fluid resuscitated
Phaeochromocytoma
Tachyarrhythmias or VF

Administration
- Larger doses: 2.5–10 µg/kg/min to increase cardiac contractility
- Doses >10 µg/kg/min stimulate α receptors and may cause renal vasoconstriction
  200 mg made up to 50 ml glucose 5% or sodium chloride 0.9% (4000 µg/ml)

Dosage chart (ml/h)

Weight (kg)	Dose (µg/kg/min)				
	2.5	5.0	7.5	10	15
50	1.9	3.8	5.6	7.5	11.3
60	2.3	4.5	6.8	9.0	13.5
70	2.6	5.3	7.9	10.5	15.8
80	3.0	6.0	9.0	12.0	18.0
90	3.4	6.8	10.1	13.5	20.3
100	3.8	7.5	11.3	15	22.5
110	4.1	8.3	12.4	16.5	24.8

Give via a central vein via accurate infusion pump

1.6 mg/ml solutions may be given via a peripheral line or central line. More concentrated solutions, including the 3.2 mg/ml solution, should be given via a central line only

Reduce dosage if urine output decreases or there is increasing tachycardia or development of new arrhythmias

How not to use dopamine
Do not use a peripheral vein (risk of extravasation)
So-called 'renal dose' dopamine for renal protection (0.5–2.5 µg/kg/min) is no longer recommended (*Crit Care Med* 2008; **36**: 296–327)
Do not connect to CVP lumen used for monitoring pressure (surge of drug during flushing of line)
Incompatible with alkaline solutions, e.g. sodium bicarbonate, furosemide, phenytoin and enoximone
Discard solution if cloudy, discoloured, or >24 h old

Adverse effects
Ectopic beats
Tachycardia
Angina
Gut ischaemia
Vasoconstriction

Cautions
MAOI (reduce dose by one-tenth of usual dose)
Peripheral vascular disease (monitor any changes in colour or temperature of the skin of the extremities)
If extravasation of dopamine occurs – phentolamine 10 mg in 15 ml sodium chloride 0.9% should be infiltrated into the ischaemic area with a 23-G needle

Organ failure
May accumulate in septic shock because of ↓ hepatic function

DOPAMINE

DOPEXAMINE

Dopexamine is the synthetic analogue of dopamine. It has potent β_2 activity with one-third the potency of dopamine on dopamine 1 receptor. There is no α activity. Dopexamine increases HR and CO, causes peripheral vasodilatation, $\uparrow$ renal and splanchnic blood flow and $\downarrow$ PCWP. Current interest in dopexamine is centred on its dopaminergic and anti-inflammatory activity. The anti-inflammatory activity and improved splanchnic blood flow may be due to dopexamine's β_2 rather than DA 1 effect. The usual dose for its anti-inflammatory activity and to improve renal, mesenteric, splanchnic and hepatic blood flow is between 0.25 and 0.5 µg/kg/min. In comparison with other inotropes, dopexamine causes less increase in myocardial oxygen consumption.

Uses
To improve renal, mesenteric, splanchnic and hepatic blood flow
Short-term treatment of acute heart failure

Contraindications
Concurrent MAOI administration
Left ventricular outlet obstruction (HOCM, aortic stenosis)
Phaeochromocytoma

Administration
Correction of hypovolaemia before starting dopexamine

• Dose: start at 0.25 µg/kg/min, increasing up to 6 µg/kg/min

Titrate according to patient's response: HR, rhythm, BP, urine output and, whenever possible, cardiac output
50 mg made up to 50 ml glucose 5% or sodium chloride 0.9% (1000 µg/ml)

Dosage chart (ml/h)

Weight (kg)	Dose (µg/kg/min)				
	0.25	0.5	1	2	3
50	0.8	1.5	3.0	6.0	9.0
60	0.9	1.8	3.6	7.2	10.8
70	1.1	2.1	4.2	8.4	12.6
80	1.2	2.4	4.8	9.6	14.4
90	1.4	2.7	5.4	10.8	16.2
100	1.5	3.0	6.0	12.0	18.0
110	1.7	3.3	6.6	13.2	19.8
120	1.8	3.6	7.2	14.4	21.6

D

How not to use dopexamine

Do not connect to CVP lumen used for monitoring pressure (surge of drug during flushing of line)

Incompatible with alkaline solutions, e.g. sodium bicarbonate, frusemide, phenytoin and enoximone

Adverse effects

Dose-related increases in HR
Hypotension
Angina
Hypokalaemia
Hyperglycaemia

Cautions

Thrombocytopenia (a further decrease may occur)
IHD (especially following acute MI)

DOPEXAMINE

ENOXAPARIN

Enoxaparin is a widely used low molecular weight heparin (LMWH), similar to dalteparin.

The incidence of bleeding is similar between LMWHs and unfractionated heparin. The incidence of immune-mediated thrombocytopenia is about 2–3% of patients treated with unfractionated heparin. LMWHs are preferred over unfractionated heparin because they are as effective, simplify treatment (usually once-daily dosing, no IV cannulation), have a lower risk of heparin-induced thrombocytopenia and monitoring is not required.

Uses
Peri- and post-operative surgical thomboprophylaxis
Medically acutely ill thomboprophylaxis
Treatment of DVT, pulmonary embolism or both
Unstable angina
Prevention of clotting in extracorporeal circuits

Contraindications
Generalised bleeding tendencies
Acute GI ulcer
Cerebral haemorrhage
Sub-acute endocarditis
Heparin-induced immune thrombocytopenia
Injuries to and operations on the CNS, eyes and ears
Known haemorrhagic diathesis
Hypersensitivity to enoxaparin or other LMWHs and/or heparins

Administration
Peri- and post-operative surgical prophylaxis – moderate risk

- 20 mg daily SC

  If CC <30 ml/min, 20 mg daily SC

Peri- and post-operative surgical prophylaxis – high risk

- 40 mg daily SC

  If CC <30 ml/min, 20 mg daily SC
  Treatment of DVT and pulmonary embolus or both
  Start enoxaparin with oral warfarin (as soon as possible) until INR in therapeutic range

- 1.5 mg/kg once daily SC

  If CC <30 ml/min, 1 mg/kg once daily SC

Acute coronary syndrome:
- 1 mg/kg 12 hourly SC, recommended treatment period up to 8 days

  If CC <30 ml/min, 1 mg/kg once-daily SC

Concomitant treatment with low–dose aspirin
Monitor: platelets
APTT monitoring is not usually required
In overdose, 1 mg enoxaparin is inhibited by 1 mg protamine

Adverse effects
Subcutaneous haematoma at injection site
Bleeding at high doses, e.g., anti–Factor Xa levels greater than 1.5 iu/ml, however at recommended doses bleeding rarely occurs
Transient increase in liver enzymes (ALT) but no clinical significance has been demonstrated
Rarely thrombocytopenia
Rarely hypoaldosteronism resulting in increased plasma potassium particularly in chronic renal failure and diabetes mellitus

How not to use enoxaparin
Not to be used for patients with heparin–induced thrombocytopenia

Renal replacement therapy
Treatment doses of low molecular weight heparins are generally avoided in RRT, since anti–Xa monitoring is required to use safely. Thus generally, use of unfractionated heparin is preferred. However for thromboprophylactic doses it appears safe to use enoxaparin 20 mg SC once daily

E

ENOXIMONE

Enoximone is a selective phosphodiesterase III inhibitor resulting in ↑ CO, and ↓ PCWP and SVR, without significant ↑ in HR and myocardial oxygen consumption. It has a long half-life and haemodynamic effects can persist for 8–10 h after the drug is stopped.

Uses
Severe congestive cardiac failure
Low cardiac output states (± dobutamine)

Contraindications
Severe aortic or pulmonary stenosis (exaggerated hypotension)
HOCM (exaggerated hypotension)

Administration
- IV infusion: 0.5–1.0 mg/kg (this dose can be omitted as can cause hypotension), then 5–20 µg/kg/min maintenance

Requires direct arterial BP monitoring
Adjustment of the infusion rate should be made according to haemodynamic response
Total dose in 24 h should not >24 mg/kg
Available in 20-ml ampoules containing 100 mg enoximone (5 mg/ml)
Dilute this 20 ml solution with 20 ml sodium chloride 0.9% giving a solution containing enoximone 2.5 mg/ml

How not to use enoximone
Glucose 5% or contact with glass may result in crystal formation
Do not dilute with very alkaline solution (incompatible with all catecholamines in solution)

Adverse effects
Hypotension
Arrhythmias

Cautions
In septic shock enoximone can cause prolonged hypotension

Organ failure
Renal: reduce dose

Renal replacement therapy
No further dose modification is required during renal replacement therapy

ENOXIMONE

EPOETIN

E

Epoetin (recombinant human erythropoetin) is available as epoetin alpha and beta. Both are similar in clinical efficacy and can be used interchangeably.

Uses
Anaemia associated with erythropoetin deficiency in chronic renal failure
Severe anaemia due to blood loss in Jehovah's Witness (unlicensed)

Contraindications
Uncontrolled hypertension
Anaemia due to iron, folic acid or vitamin B_{12} deficiency

Administration
- Chronic renal failure

  Aim to increase haemoglobin concentration at rate not >2 g/100 ml per month to stable level of 10–12 g/100 ml
  SC (maximum 1 ml per injection site) or IV given over 3–5 min
  Initially 50 units/kg three times weekly increased according to response in steps of 25 units/kg at intervals of 4 weeks
  Maintenance dose (when haemoglobin 10–12 g/100 ml) 50–300 units/kg weekly in 2–3 divided doses

- Severe anaemia due to blood loss in Jehovah's Witness

  150–300 units/kg daily SC until desired haemoglobin reached
  Supplementary iron (e.g. ferrous sulphate 200 mg PO) and O_2 is mandatory
  Monitor: BP, haemoglobin, serum ferritin, platelet and electrolytes

How not to use epoetin
Avoid contact of reconstituted injection with glass; use only plastic materials

Adverse effects
Dose-dependent increase in BP and platelet count
Flu-like symptoms (reduced if IV given over 5 min)
Shunt thrombosis
Hyperkalaemia
Increase in plasma urea, creatinine and phosphate
Convulsions
Skin reactions
Palpebral oedema
Myocardial infarction
Anaphylaxis

EPOETIN

E

Cautions
Hypertension (stop if uncontrolled)
Ischaemic vascular disease
Thrombocytosis (monitor platelet count for first 8 weeks)
Epilepsy
Malignant disease
Chronic liver disease

EPOPROSTENOL (Flolan)

Epoprostenol has a half-life of only 3 min. When given intravenously, it is a potent vasodilator and therefore its side-effects include flushing, headaches and hypotension. Epoprostenol may be used instead of or in addition to heparin during haemofiltration to inhibit platelet aggregation. The dose is dictated by clinical need and filter life (ideally at least 2–3 days).

Uses

Haemofiltration (unlicensed), as an alternative to unfractionated heparin in heparin-induced thrombocytopenia or in addition to heparin if filter life is short

ARDS/Pulmonary hypertension (unlicensed)
Peripheral insufficiency

Administration

• Haemofiltration

Infusion into extracorporeal circuit 2–10 ng/kg/min, start 1 h before haemofiltration. For peripheral insufficiency, administer this dose IV. Available in vials containing 500 μg (500 000 nanograms) epoprostenol. Reconstitute the powder with 10 ml of the diluent provided. Once powder has dissolved, withdraw the contents from the vial and inject into the remaining diluents (40 ml) in the large vial. This results in a concentrated solution of epoprostenol. Connect the filter provided to a needle and withdraw 50 ml of the solution into a 50-ml syringe

Dosage chart (ml/h)

Weight (kg)	Dose (ng/kg/min)								
	2	3	4	5	6	7	8	9	10
50	0.6	0.9	1.2	1.5	1.8	2.1	2.4	2.7	3.0
60	0.7	1.1	1.4	1.8	2.2	2.5	2.9	3.2	3.6
70	0.8	1.3	1.7	2.1	2.5	2.9	3.4	3.8	4.2
80	1.0	1.4	1.9	2.4	2.9	3.4	3.8	4.3	4.8
90	1.1	1.6	2.2	2.7	3.2	3.8	4.3	4.9	5.4
100	1.2	1.8	2.4	3.0	3.6	4.2	4.8	5.4	6.0

• ARDS/pulmonary hypertension

Nebulised (unlicensed): 1–20 ng/kg/min of the reconstituted powder (500 μg epoprostenol reconstituted with the 50 ml diluent provided) into ventilator circuit via compressed air nebuliser systems

E

How not to use epoprostenol
To avoid systemic side-effects in CVVH, it may be preferable to administer epoprostenol into the extracorporeal circuit and not into the patient

The integrated syringe pump on some haemofiltration machines may not be accurate enough to deliver the correct dose of epoprostenol. If so, use a stand-alone syringe pump.

Adverse effects
Flushing
Headaches
Hypotension
Bradycardia

Cautions
Epoprostenol may potentiate heparin effects

ERYTHROMYCIN

Erythromycin has an antibacterial spectrum similar but not identical to that of penicillin; it is thus an alternative in penicillin-allergic patients. Resistance rates in Gram +ve organisms limit its use for severe soft tissue infections. Erythromycin has also been used as a prokinetic in gastric stasis and in aiding the passage of fine-bore feeding tube beyond the pylorus. Erythromycin is an agonist at motilin receptors. Motilin is a peptide secreted in the small intestine, which induces GI contractions, so increasing gut motility. Use as a prokinetic may increase patient colonisation with resistant bacterial species, including MRSA.

Uses
Alternative to penicillin (in patients with genuine penicillin allergy)
Community-acquired pneumonia, particularly caused by atypical organisms
Infective exacerbations of COPD
Legionnaires' disease
Pharyngeal and sinus infections
As a prokinetic (unlicensed)

Administration
- IV infusion: 0.5–1.0 g 6 hourly

  Reconstitute with 20 ml WFI, shake well, then further dilute in 250 ml sodium chloride 0.9% given over 1 hour
  CC >10 ml/min normal dose
  CC <10 ml/min 50–75% of dose, maximum 2 g daily in split doses

- As a prokinetic: 125 mg 6 hourly PO/NG, 125–250 mg 6–12 hourly IV

How not to use erythromycin
IV bolus is not recommended
No other diluent (apart from WFI) should be used for the initial reconstitution
Do not use concurrently with simvastatin (myopathy) or sertindole (ventricular arrhythmias)

Adverse effects
Gastrointestinal intolerance
Hypersensitivity reactions
Reversible hearing loss with large doses
Cholestatic jaundice if given >14 days
Prolongation of QT interval

E

Cautions
↑ plasma levels of alfentanil, carbamazepine, ciclosporin, midazolam, phenytoin, theophylline, valproate, warfarin and zopiclone
Severe renal impairment (ototoxicity)
Hepatic disease

Organ failure
Renal: reduce dose

Renal replacement therapy
No further dose modification is required during renal replacement therapy

ERYTHROMYCIN

ESMOLOL (Brevibloc)

E

Esmolol is a relatively cardioselective β-blocker with a rapid onset and a very short duration of action. Esmolol is metabolised by esterases in the red blood cells and the elimination half-life is about 9 min. It is used IV for the short-term treatment of supraventricular arrhythmias, sinus tachycardia or hypertension and is particularly useful in the peri-operative period.

Uses
AF
Atrial flutter
Sinus tachycardia
Hypertension

Contraindications
Unstable asthma
Severe bradycardia
Sick sinus syndrome
Second- or third–degree AV block
Uncontrolled heart failure
Hypotension

Administration
- IV bolus: 80 mg loading bolus over 15–30 s, followed by IV infusion
- IV infusion: 50–200 µg/kg/min (210–840 or 21–84 ml/h in a 70-kg individual)

  Available in 10-ml vial containing 100 mg esmolol (10 mg/ml) to be used undiluted and 10 ml ampoule containing 2.5 g esmolol (250 mg/ml) requiring dilution to 10 mg/ml solution. Dilute 5 g (two ampoules) in 500 ml sodium chloride 0.9% or glucose 5% (10 mg/ml)

How not to use esmolol
Not compatible with sodium bicarbonate
Esmolol 2.5-g ampoules must be diluted before infusion

Cautions
Asthma

Adverse effects
Bradycardia
Heart failure
Hypotension
These side-effects should resolve within 30 min of discontinuing infusion

FENTANYL

Fentanyl is 100 times as potent as morphine. Its onset of action is within 1–2 min after IV injection and a peak effect within 4–5 min. Duration of action after a single bolus is 20 min. The context sensitive half-life following IV infusion is prolonged because of its large volume of distribution.

Uses
Analgesia

Contraindications
Airway obstruction

Administration
• For sedation
   IV infusion: 1–5 μg/kg/h
• During anaesthesia
   IV bolus:
   • 1–3 μg/kg with spontaneous ventilation
   • 5–10 μg/kg with IPPV
   • 7–10 μg/kg to obtund pressor response of laryngoscopy
   • Up to 100 μg/kg for cardiac surgery

How not to use fentanyl
In combination with an opioid partial agonist, e.g. buprenorphine (antagonises opioid effects)

Adverse effects
Respiratory depression and apnoea
Bradycardia and hypotension
Nausea and vomiting
Delayed gastric emptying
Reduce intestinal mobility
Biliary spasm
Constipation
Urinary retention
Chest wall rigidity (may interfere with ventilation)
Muscular rigidity and hypotension more common after high dosage

Cautions
Enhanced sedation and respiratory depression from interaction with:

• benzodiazepines
• antidepressants
• anti-psychotics

Head injury and neurosurgical patients (may exacerbate ↑ ICP as a result of ↑ $PaCO_2$)

Organ failure
Respiratory: ↑ respiratory depression
Hepatic: enhanced and prolonged sedative effect

FLUCLOXACILLIN

A derivative of the basic penicillin structure which has stability to the staphylococcal penicillinase found in most *Staphylococcus aureus* isolates. Generally less active than benzylpenicillin against other Gram +ve organisms. Strains which express resistance are designated methicillin resistant and are known as MRSAs.

Uses
Infections due to penicillinase–producing staphylococci (except MRSA):

- cellulitis
- wound infection
- endocarditis
- adjunct in pneumonia
- osteomyelitis
- septic arthritis

Contraindications
Penicillin hypersensitivity

Administration
IV: 0.25–2 g 6 hourly, depending on the severity of infection. For endocarditis (in combination with another antibiotic), 2 g 6 hourly, increasing to 2 g 4 hourly if over 85 kg

Reconstitute with 20 ml WFI, given over 3–5 min

Infection	Dose (g)	Interval (h)
Mild–moderate	0.25–0.5	6
Moderate–serious	1–2	6
Life-threatening	2	6

In renal impairment:
CC >10 ml/min dose as per normal renal function
CC <10 ml/min dose as in normal renal function up to a total daily dose of 4 g

How not to use flucloxacillin
Not for intrathecal use (encephalopathy)
Do not mix in the same syringe with an aminoglycoside (efficacy of aminoglycoside reduced)

Adverse effects
Hypersensitivity
Haemolytic anaemia
Transient neutropenia and thrombocytopenia
Cholestatic jaundice and hepatitis

- ↑ risk with treatment >2 weeks and increasing age
- may occur up to several weeks after stopping treatment

Cautions
Liver failure (worsening of LFTs)

Organ failure
Renal: reduce dose
Hepatic: avoid

Renal replacement therapy
No further dose modification is required during renal replacement therapy

FLUCONAZOLE

F

Antifungal active against *Candida albicans*, *Candida tropicalis*, *Candida parapsilosis* and cryptococcus. Variable activity against *Candida glabrata* and poor activity for *Candida krusei*. It is rapidly and completely absorbed orally. Oral and IV therapy equally effective; IV for patients unable to take orally. Widely distributed in tissues and fluids. Excreted unchanged in urine.

Uses
- Local or systemic candidiasis
- Cryptococcal infections – usually follow-on therapy after amphotericin

Administration
- Oropharyngeal candidiasis

    Orally: 50–100 mg daily for 7–14 days

- Oesophageal candidiasis or candiduria

    Orally: 50–100 mg daily for 14–30 days

- Systemic candidiasis or cryptococcal infections

    IV infusion: 400 mg daily, consider higher doses for less susceptible *Candida* isolates
    Infusion rate 10–20 mg/min

Continued according to response (at least 6–8 weeks for cryptococcal meningitis; often longer)

In renal impairment:
    10 ml/min normal dose
    <10 ml/min use 50% of normal dose

How not to use fluconazole
Avoid concurrent use with astemizole or terfenadine (arrhythmias)

Adverse effects
Rash
Pruritis
Nausea, vomiting, diarrhoea
Raised liver enzymes
Hypersensitivity

Cautions
Renal/hepatic impairment
May increase concentrations of ciclosporin, phenytoin, warfarin, midazolam, theophylline and tacrolimus. Possible increased risk of myopathy with simvastatin and atorvastatin

Organ failure
Renal: reduce dose

Renal replacement therapy

CVVH dialysed, no dose reduction needed, if high filtration rates are used or haemodiafiltration then higher doses may be needed, e.g. 600–800 mg daily. HD dialysed, dose as in CC < 10 ml/min, i.e. use half normal dose or 100% of dose three times per week after dialysis. PD dialysed, use 50% of normal dose. Three hours of HD have been shown to reduce fluconazole plasma levels by 50%.

FLUMAZENIL

A competitive antagonist at the benzodiazepine receptor. It has a short duration of action (20 min).

Uses
To facilitate weaning from ventilation in patients sedated with benzo-diazepine
In the management of benzodiazepine overdose
As a diagnostic test for the cause of prolonged sedation

Contraindications
Tricyclic antidepressant and mixed-drug overdose (fits)
Patients on long-term benzodiazepine therapy (withdrawal)
Epileptic patients on benzodiazepines (fits)
Patients with raised ICP (further increase in ICP)

Administration
• IV bolus: 200 μg, repeat at 1 min intervals until desired response, up to a total dose of 2 mg

If re-sedation occurs, repeat dose every 20 min

How not to use flumazenil
Ensure effects of neuromuscular blockade reversed before using fluma-zenil

Adverse effects
Dizziness
Agitation
Arrhythmias
Hypertension
Epileptic fits

Cautions
Re-sedation – requires prolonged monitoring if long-acting benzodi-azepines have been taken

Organ failure
Hepatic: reduced elimination

FONDAPARINUX (Arixtra)

Fondaparinux is a synthetic pentasaccharide that binds to anti-thrombin and enhances the inactivation of factor Xa without interaction with factor II or platelets. It is licensed for thromboprophylaxis and full anticoagulation, including acute coronary syndrome. It can be used in patients with heparin-induced thrombocytopenia (HIT). The main critical care use of this drug will be in HIT and in high risk post-operative patients. There is no antidote to its use. It has an elimination half-life of 17–21 hours after subcutaneous injection, allowing once daily dosing. Up to 80% is excreted unmetabolised in the urine, dose reduction is required in renal impairment.

Uses

Anticoagulation in HIT
Prevention of thromboembolism (with or without HIT)
Acute coronary syndrome

Contraindications

Haemophilia and other haemorrhagic disorders
Thrombocytopenia (except HIT)
Recent cerebral haemorrhage
Severe hypertension
Active peptic ulcer (unless this is the reason for operation)
Diabetic retinopathy
Acute bacterial endocarditis
Spinal or epidural anaesthesia with treatment doses of danaparoid

Administration

- Thromboprophylaxis after surgery: 2.5 mg SC 6 hours after surgery then 2.5 mg once daily
- Thromboprophylaxis in medical patients: 2.5 mg SC once daily
- Treatment of DVT/PE

  <50 kg, 5 mg SC daily
  50–100 kg, 7.5 mg SC daily
  >100 kg, 10 mg SC daily
  Warfarin can be started at the same time as fondaparinux (fondaparinux should be continued for at least 5 days and until INR ≥2 for at least 24 hours)

- Treatment of superficial-vein thrombosis

  50 kg, 2.5 mg SC once daily for at least 30 days (max. 45 days if high risk of thromboembolic complications); treatment should be stopped 24 hours before surgery and restarted at least 6 hours post-op

- ACS: 2.5 mg SC once daily for up to 8 days (or until hospital discharge if sooner); treatment should be stopped 24 hours before CABG surgery (where possible) and restarted 48 hours post-op

F

In renal impairment
GFR ml/min

20–50	Prophylactic dose: 1.5 mg SC daily
30–70 and >100 kg	Treatment of DVT/PE: initial dose of 10 mg SC then reduce to 7.5 mg SC daily
10–20	Use with caution
<10	Use with caution

Adverse effects
Bleeding
Hypersensitivity reactions (including rash)

Renal replacement therapy
For haemofiltration, see under administration

FONDAPARINUX (Arixtra)

FUROSEMIDE

Furosemide is a widely used loop diuretic. Following an IV bolus, the diuretic effect peaks within 30 min. It produces relief of dyspnoea (by reduction in pre-load) sooner than would be expected from the diuresis. The diuretic effect is dose related. In patients with impaired renal function larger doses may be necessary.

Uses

Acute oliguric renal failure – may convert acute oliguric to nonoliguric renal failure. Other measures must be taken to ensure adequate circulating blood volume and renal perfusion pressure

Pulmonary oedema – secondary to acute left ventricular failure

Oedema – associated with congestive cardiac failure, hepatic failure and renal disease

Contraindications

Oliguria secondary to hypovolaemia

Administration

- IV bolus: 10–40 mg over 3–5 min
- IV infusion: 2–10 mg/h

For high-dose parenteral therapy (up to 1000 mg/day), dilute in 250–500 ml sodium chloride 0.9% given at a rate not >240 mg/h

How not to use furosemide

Glucose-containing fluid is not recommended as a diluent (infusion pH >5.5, otherwise may precipitate)

Do not give at >240 mg/h (transient deafness)

Adverse effects

Hyponatraemia, hypokalaemia, hypomagnesaemia

Hyperuricaemia, hyperglycaemia

Ototoxicity

Nephrotoxicity

Pancreatitis

Cautions

Amphotericin (increased risk of hypokalaemia)

Aminoglycosides (increased nephrotoxicity and ototoxicity)

Digoxin toxicity (due to hypokalaemia)

Organ failure

Renal: may need to increase dose for effect

Renal replacement therapy

No further dose modification is required during renal replacement therapy

GANCICLOVIR (Cymevene)

Ganciclovir is related to aciclovir but is more active against cytomega-lovirus (CMV). It is also more toxic. It causes profound myelo-suppression when given with zidovudine; the two should not be given together particularly during initial ganciclovir therapy.

Uses
CMV infections in immunocompromised patients
Prevention of CMV infection during immunosuppression following organ transplantation

Contraindications
Hypersensitivity to ganciclovir and aciclovir
Abnormally low neutrophil counts

Administration
* IV infusion: 5 mg/kg 12 hourly, given over 1 h through filter provided

  Though not cytotoxic, this product should preferably be made up aseptically as it is myelosuppressive. Reconstitute the 500 mg pow-der with 10 ml WFI, then dilute with 50–100 ml sodium chloride 0.9% or glucose 5%
  Wear polythene gloves and safety glasses when preparing solution
  Duration of treatment: 7–14 days for prevention and 14–21 days for treatment
  Ensure adequate hydration

Monitor: FBC
   U&E
   LFT
In renal impairment:

CC (ml/min)	Dose (mg/kg)	Interval (h)
70	5.0	12
50–69	2.5	12
25–49	2.5	24
0–24	1.25	24

Adverse effects
Leucopenia
Thrombocytopenia
Anaemia
Fever
Rash
Abnormal LFT

Cautions
History of cytopenia, low platelet count
Concurrent use of myelosuppressants
Renal impairment

Renal replacement therapy
The major route of clearance of ganciclovir is by glomerular filtration of the unchanged drug. CVVH dialysed, dependent on clearance rate as described in Short Notes Renal Replacement Therapy (p. 300–303) and CC table above. HD dialysed, 1.25 mg/kg every day post-dialysis on dialysis days. PD dialysable, 1.25 mg/kg IV every 24 hours

GENTAMICIN

This is the aminoglycoside most commonly used in the UK. It is effective against Gram −ve organisms such as *E. coli*, *Klebsiella* spp., *Proteus* spp., *Serratia* spp. and *Pseudomonas aeruginosa*. It is also active against *Staphylococcus aureus*. It is inactive against anaerobes and has poor activity against all streptococci including *Strep. pyogenes and Strep. pneumoniae*, and *Enterococus* spp. When given in combination with a penicillin, excellent synergy is achieved against most strains of *streptococci* and *enterococci*. When used for the 'blind' therapy of undiagnosed serious infections it is usually given with a penicillin and metronidazole, if indicated (e.g. abdominal sepsis).

It is not appreciably absorbed orally and is renally excreted unchanged. In renal impairment the half-life is prolonged. Most side-effects are related to sustained high trough concentrations. Efficacy, on the other hand, is related to peak concentrations that are well in excess of the minimum inhibitory concentration of the infecting organism. Plasma concentration monitoring is essential.

High-dose single daily dosing of aminoglycosides has become more popular. It ensures that target peak concentrations are achieved in all patients and may also be less nephrotoxic. It also makes monitoring of gentamicin levels easier.

Uses
Sepsis of unknown origin (with a penicillin and/or metronidazole)
Intra-abdominal infections (with a penicillin and metronidazole)
Acute pyelonephritis (with ampicillin)
Infective endocarditis (beta lactam)
Hospital-acquired pneumonia (with a third-generation cephalosporin)
Severe infections due to *P. aeruginosa* (with ceftazidime or piperacillin/tazobactam)
Enterococcal infections (with amoxicillin)
Febrile neutropenia (with ceftazidime or piperacillin/tazobactam)

Contraindications
Pregnancy
Myasthenia gravis

G

Administration

- Rapid IV bolus: 1–1.5 mg/kg IV 8 hourly

In renal impairment:

CC (ml/min)	Dose (mg/kg)	Interval (h)
20–50	1.5	12–24
10–20	1.0–1.5	12–24
<10	1.0	24–48

Monitor plasma level (p. 250): adjust dose/interval accordingly

- High dose single daily dosing protocol

  Avoid this regimen in renal replacement therapy or if the CC <20 ml/min

IV infusion: 7 mg/kg in 50 ml glucose 5% or sodium chloride 0.9% given over 1 hour. For obese patients lean body weight should be used (see Appendix D). The interval is then decided after referring to the Hartford nomogram (developed and validated by DP Nicolau et al., Division of Infectious Diseases, Hartford Hospital, Hartford, Connecticut, USA). A blood level is taken after the first dose to determine subsequent dosing interval. Alternative nomograms have also been developed for 5 mg/kg dosing. Do not use this nomogram for any other single dosing protocol

Monitoring: Take a single blood sample at any time 6–14 hours after the *start* of an IV infusion. It is essential that the *exact* time is recorded accurately

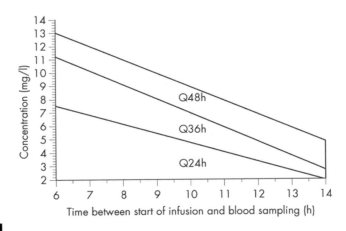

Time between start of infusion and blood sampling (h)

GENTAMICIN

G

Evaluate the nomogram. If the level lies in the area designated Q24, Q36 or Q48, the interval should be every 24, 36 or 48 hourly respectively. Frequency of repeat levels depends on underlying renal function

If the point is on the line, choose the longer interval. If the dosing interval is greater than 48 hours, an alternative antibiotic should be used. Single daily dosing should not be used for children, pregnant women, burns patients, infective endocarditis and patients with significant pre-existing renal impairment. It should be used with caution in very septic patients with incipient renal failure

How not to use gentamicin
Do not mix in a syringe with penicillins and cephalosporins (aminoglycosides inactivated)

Adverse effects
Nephrotoxicity − ↑ risk with amphotericin, bumetanide, furosemide, vancomycin and lithium

Ototoxicity − ↑ risk with pre-existing renal insufficiency, elderly, bumetanide and furosemide
Prolonged neuromuscular blockade − may be clinically significant in patients being weaned from mechanical ventilation

Cautions
Renal impairment (reduce dose)
Concurrent use of:

- amphotericin − ↑ nephrotoxicity
- bumetanide, furosemide − ↑ ototoxicity
- neuromuscular blockers − prolonged muscle weakness

Organ failure
Renal: increased plasma concentration − ↑ ototoxicity and nephrotoxicity

Renal replacement therapy
CVVH dialysed dependent on clearance rate as described in Short Notes Renal Replacement Therapy (p. 300–303) and CC table given previously. Some units dose 3–5 mg/kg daily and monitor levels. Levels must be monitored, and dose and interval adjusted accordingly. HD/PD dialysed, dose as in CC 5–10 ml/min, i.e. 2 mg/kg every 48–72 hours; for HD, dose post-dialysis. One hour peak levels should not exceed 10 mg/ml and pre-dose trough should be <2 mg/l

GLUTAMINE

Glutamine is primarily synthesised in skeletal muscle and is the most abundant amino acid. It is a major metabolic fuel for the enterocytes in the gut mucosa. Glutamine is also required for lymphocyte and macrophage function, and is a precursor for nucleotide synthesis. Glutathione is a product of glutamine metabolism, and has an important role as an antioxidant. Although not regarded as an essential amino acid, it becomes conditionally essential in catabolic states. Surgery, trauma or sepsis decreases plasma concentrations. Some studies have shown that glutamine-supplemented enteral feeds improve nitrogen balance, reduce infections and length of hospital stay. This may, at least in part, be explained by the reduced bacterial translocation. However, none of these studies has shown improved survival when compared with standard feeds (p. 286).

Uses
Immunonutrition – to maintain gut integrity and prevent bacterial translocation during critical illness

Administration
Orally: 5 g 6 hourly
Dissolve the 5-g sachet in 20 ml WFI

Cautions
Phenylketonuria (contains aspartame)

GLYCEROL SUPPOSITORY

G

Glycerol suppositories act as a rectal stimulant by virtue of the mildly irritant action of glycerol.

Uses
Constipation

Contraindications
Intestinal obstruction

Administration
PR: 4 g suppository moistened with water before insertion

How not to use glycerol suppository
Not for prolonged use

Adverse effects
Abdominal discomfort

Cautions
Prolonged use (atonic colon and hypokalaemia)

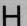

HALOPERIDOL

A butyrophenone with longer duration of action than droperidol. It has anti-emetic and neuroleptic effects with minimal cardiovascular and respiratory effects. It is a mild α-blocker and may cause hypotension in the presence of hypovolaemia.

Uses
Acute agitation and delirium

Contraindications
QT prolongation, torsades de pointe, ventricular arrhythmias, agitation caused by hypoxia, hypokalaemia or a full bladder
Parkinson's disease

Administration
- IV bolus: 2.5–5 mg
- IV infusion: 30 mg in 50 ml of glucose 5% at a rate of 0–10 mg/h (unlicensed administration)
- IM: 5–10 mg

Up to every 4–8 h

How not to use haloperidol
Hypotension resulting from haloperidol should not be treated with adrenaline as a further decrease in BP may result

Adverse effects
Extra-pyramidal movements
Neuroleptic malignant syndrome (treat with dantrolene)
Prolongation of QT interval

Cautions
Concurrent use of other CNS depressants (enhanced sedation)

Organ failure
CNS: sedative effects increased
Hepatic: can precipitate coma
Renal: increased cerebral sensitivity

Renal replacement therapy
No further dose modification is required during renal replacement therapy

HEPARIN

Uses
Prophylaxis of DVT and PE
Treatment of DVT and PE
Extracorporeal circuits

Contraindications
Haemophilia and other haemorrhagic disorders
Peptic ulcer
Cerebral haemorrhage
Severe hypertension
Severe liver disease (including oesophageal varices)
Severe renal failure
Thrombocytopenia
Hypersensitivity to heparin

Administration
- Prophylaxis of DVT and PE

  SC: 5000 units 8–12 hourly until patient is ambulant

- Treatment of DVT and PE

  IV: Loading dose of 5000 units followed by continuous infusion of 1000–2000 units/h
  20,000 units heparin in 20 ml undiluted (1000 units/ml). Check APTT 6 h after loading dose and adjust rate to keep APTT between 1.5 and 2.5 times normal (or 2–3 depending on laboratory reference range)

Unfractionated heparin nomogram:

APTT ratio	Infusion rate change (NB: do NOT use this for heparin infusion post-acute MI)
>7	Stop for 1 h, recheck APTT ratio and then reduce by 500 units/h
5.1–7.0	Reduce by 500 units/h
4.1–5.0	Reduce by 300 units/h
3.1–4.0	Reduce by 100 units/h
2.6–3.0	Reduce by 50 units/h
1.5–2.5	NO CHANGE
1.2–1.4	Increase by 200 units/h
<1.2	Consider 2500 units IV bolus, increase by 400 units/h

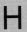

Start oral warfarin as soon as the patient is stable

- Haemofiltration

  1000 units to run through the system. Then a bolus of 1500–3000 units injected into the pre-filter port, followed by 5–10 units/kg/h infused into the pre-filter port

  Dose is dictated by clinical need and filter life (ideally at least 2–3 days)

Adverse effects
Haemorrhage
Skin necrosis
Thrombocytopenia
Hypersensitivity
Osteoporosis after prolonged use

Cautions
Hepatic impairment (avoid if severe)

HYDRALAZINE (Apresoline)

Hydralazine lowers the BP by reducing arterial resistance through a direct relaxation of arteriolar smooth muscle. This effect is limited by reflex tachycardia and so it is best combined with a β-blocker. Metabolism occurs by hepatic acetylation, the rate of which is genetically determined. Fast acetylators show a reduced therapeutic effect until the enzyme system is saturated.

Uses
All grades of hypertension
Pre-eclampsia

Contraindications
Systemic lupus erythematosus
Dissecting aortic aneurysm
Right ventricular failure due to pulmonary hypertension (cor pulmonale)
Severe tachycardia and heart failure with a high cardiac output state, e.g. thyrotoxicosis
Severe aortic outflow obstruction (aortic stenosis, mitral stenosis, constrictive pericarditis)

Administration
- IV bolus: 10–20 mg over 3–5 min

  Reconstitute the ampoule containing 20 mg powder with 1 ml WFI, further dilute with 10 ml sodium chloride 0.9% give over 3–5 min
  Expect to see response after 20 min
  Repeat after 20–30 min as necessary

- IV infusion: 2–15 mg/h

  Reconstitute three ampoules (60 mg) of hydralazine with 1 ml WFI each. Make up to 60 ml with sodium chloride 0.9% (1 mg/ml)
  Give at a rate between 2 and 15 mg/h depending on the BP and pulse
  Rapid acetylators may require higher doses

- PO: hypertension 25 mg twice daily (up to 50 mg twice daily)

  Heart failure 25 mg 6–8 hourly, increased every 2 days to 50–75 mg 6 hourly

How not to use hydralazine
Do not dilute in fluids containing glucose (causes breakdown of hydralazine)

Adverse effects
Headache
Tachycardia
Hypotension

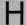

Myocardial ischaemia

Sodium and fluid retention, producing oedema and reduced urinary volume (prevented by concomitant use of a diuretic)

Lupus erythematosus (commoner if slow acetylator status, women and if treatment >6 months at doses >100 mg daily)

Cautions

Cerebrovascular disease

Cardiac disease (angina, immediately post-MI)

Use with other antihypertensives and nitrate drugs may produce additive hypotensive effects

Organ failure

Hepatic: prolonged effect

Renal: increased hypotensive effect (start with small dose)

HYDROCORTISONE

In the critically ill patient, adrenocortical insufficiency should be considered when an inappropriate amount of inotropic support is required. Baseline cortisol levels and short synacthen test do not predict response to steroid. In patients who demonstrate a normal short synacthen test, but yet show a dramatic response to steroid, it is possible that the abnormality lies in altered receptor function or glucocorticoid resistance rather than abnormality of the adrenal axis. Baseline cortisol levels and short synacthen test are worthwhile to assess hypothalamic–pituitary–adrenal axis dysfunction versus steroid unresponsiveness.

Available as the sodium succinate or the phosphate ester

Uses
Adrenal insufficiency (primary or secondary)
Prolonged resistant vasopressor dependent shock
Severe bronchospasm
Hypersensitivity reactions (p. 259)
Fibroproliferative phase of ARDS (unlicensed)
Adjunct in *Pneumocystis carinii* pneumonia (see co-trimoxazole and pentamidine)

Contraindications
Systemic infection (unless specific anti-microbial therapy given)

Administration
• Adrenal insufficiency

Major surgery or stress: IV 100–500 mg 6–8 hourly
Minor surgery: IV 50 mg 8–12 hourly
Reduce by 25% per day until normal oral steroids resumed or maintained on 20 mg in the morning and 10 mg in the evening IV

• Prolonged resistant vasopressor-dependent shock

Initial dose 50 mg IV bolus, 6 hourly for 5 days, then 50 mg 12 hourly for 3 days, then 50 mg daily for 3 days, then stop or 50 mg IV bolus followed by infusion of 10 mg/h for up to 48 hours

• Fibroproliferative phase of ARDS

IV infusion: 100–200 mg 6 hourly for up to 3 days, then dose reduced gradually

• Adjunct in *Pneumocystis carinii* pneumonia (see co-trimoxazole and pentamidine)

IV: 100 mg 6 hourly for 5 days, then dose reduced to complete 21 days of treatment
The steroid should be started at the same time as the co-trimoxazole or pentamidine and should be withdrawn before the antibiotic treatment is complete

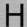

Reconstitute 100 mg powder with 2 ml WFI. Further dilute 200 mg and made up to 40 ml with sodium chloride 0.9% or glucose 5% (5 mg/ml)

How not to use hydrocortisone
Do not stop abruptly (adrenocortical insufficiency)

Adverse effects
Perineal irritation may follow IV administration of the phosphate ester
Prolonged use may also lead to the following problems:

- increased susceptibility to infections
- impaired wound healing
- peptic ulceration
- muscle weakness (proximal myopathy)
- osteoporosis
- hyperglycaemia

Cautions
Diabetes mellitus
Concurrent use of NSAID (increased risk of GI bleeding)

HYDROCORTISONE

IMIPENEM + CILASTATIN (Primaxin)

Imipenem is given in combination with cilastatin, a specific inhibitor of the renal enzyme dehydropeptidase-1 that inactivates imipenem. Imipenem has been widely replaced by meropenem. Imipenem has an extremely wide spectrum of activity, including most aerobic and anaerobic Gram −ve, including those expressing extended spectrum beta-lactamases, and Gram +ve bacteria (but not MRSA). It has no activity against *Stenotrophomonas maltophilia*, which emerges in some patients treated with imipenem. Acquired resistance is relatively common in *P. aeruginosa* and is starting to emerge in some of the Enterobacteriaceae including *Enterobacter* spp., *Citrobacter* spp. and the Proteus group.

Uses
- Mixed aerobic/anaerobic infections
- Presumptive therapy prior to availability of sensitivities for a wide range of severe infections
- Febrile neutropenia

Contraindications
CNS infections (neurotoxicity)
Meningitis (neurotoxicity)

Administration
- IV infusion: 0.5–1 g 6–8 hourly depending on severity of infection

  Dilute with sodium chloride 0.9% or glucose 5% to a concentration of 5 mg/ml
  500 mg: add 100 ml diluent, infuse over 30 min
  1 g: add 200 ml diluent, infuse over 60 min
  Unstable at room temperature following reconstitution – use immediately

In renal impairment:

CC (ml/min)	Dose (g)	Interval (h)
31–70	0.5–1	8
21–30	0.5–1	12
<20	0.25*	12

*or 3.5 mg/kg, whichever is lower

How not to use imipenem
Not compatible with diluents containing lactate

Adverse effects
Hypersensitivity reactions
Blood disorders
Positive Coombs' test
↑ Liver function tests, serum creatinine and blood urea
Myoclonic activity
Convulsions (high doses or renal impairment)

Cautions
Hypersensitivity to penicillins and cephalosporins
Renal impairment
Elderly

Organ failure
Renal: reduce dose

Renal replacement therapy
Dependent on clearance rate as described in Short Notes Renal Replacement Therapy (p. 300–303) and CC table given previously.

IMMUNOGLOBULIN

Human normal immunoglobulin is prepared by cold alcohol fractionation of pooled plasma from over 1000 donations. Individual donor units of plasma are screened for hepatitis B surface antigen (HBsAg) and for the presence of antibodies to human immunodeficiency virus type 1 (HIV-1), HIV-2 or hepatitis C virus (HCV) which, combined with careful donor selection, minimises the risk of viral transmission. In addition, the testing for HBsAg, HIV-1, HIV-2 and HCV antibodies is repeated on the plasma pools.

Uses
Guillain–Barré syndrome
Weakness during exacerbations in myasthenia gravis (unlicensed)
Toxic shock syndromes (unlicensed)

Contraindications
Patients with known class-specific antibody to IgA (risk of anaphylactoid reactions)

IV Ig administration and thromboembolic events such as myocardial infarction, stroke, pulmonary embolism and deep vein thrombosis, which is assumed to be related to a relative increase in blood viscosity

Administration
- For Guillain–Barré syndrome and myasthenia gravis

  IV infusion: 0.4 g/kg IV daily for 5 consecutive days. Repeat at 4-week intervals if necessary
  Patient treated for the first time: give at rate of 30 ml/h, if no adverse effects occur within 15 min, increase rate to maximum of 150 ml/h
  Subsequent infusions: give at rate of 100 ml/h

- Toxic shock: 1 g/kg day 1, then 0.5 g/kg for days 2 and 3 (this regimen was used by Darenberg J., et al. *CID* 2003; **37**: 333–40)

Immunoglobulin distributes poorly into adipose tissue; for patients with BMI ≥30 kg/m^2 or if actual weight >20% more than IBW (ideal body weight), consider using adjusted body weight dosing of immunoglobulin, rounded to the nearest 10% of the calculated dose (http://www.nsd.scot.nhs.uk/Documents/clinimmumoMarch12.pdf)

IBW for males = 50 + [2.3 × (height in inches − 60)]

IBW for female = 45.5 + [2.3 × (height in inches − 60)]

Adjusted body weight (kg): = IBW + 0.4 [actual body weight (kg) − IBW]

Certain immunoglobulins require refrigeration. These should be allowed to reach room temperature before administration. Once reconstituted, avoid shaking the bottle (risk of foaming). The solution should be used only if it is clear, and given without delay

How not to use immunoglobulins

Should not be mixed with any other drug and should always be given through a separate infusion line

Live virus vaccines (except yellow fever) should be given at least 3 weeks before or 3 months after an injection of normal immunoglobulin. Doses are not necessarily interchangeable between different IVIG products, check product literature on www.medicines.org.uk

Adverse effects

Chills

Fever

Transient ↑ serum creatinine

↑ thromboembolic events, e.g. MI, stroke, PE and DVT – assumed to be related to a relative ↑ in blood viscosity

Anaphylaxis (rare)

INSULIN

Insulin plays a key role in the regulation of carbohydrate, fat and protein metabolism. Hyperglycaemia and insulin resistance are common in critically ill patients, even if they have not previously had diabetes. Two studies (Van den Berghe G, et al. *N Engl J Med* 2001; **345**: 1349–67 and Van den Berghe G, et al. *N Engl J Med* 2006; **354**: 449–61) have shown that tight control of blood glucose levels (between 4.4 and 6.1 mmol/l) reduces mortality among longer stay (≥3 days) adult intensive care patients. The incidence of complications such as septicaemia, acute renal failure and critical illness polyneuropathy may also be reduced. In practice, however, many centres have found this tight control problematic, with increased risks of hypoglycaemic events. Indeed the NICE-SUGAR study (*N Engl J Med* 2009; **360**: 1283–97) reported a higher mortality with tight glucose control.

Uses
- Hyperglycaemia
- Tight glucose control
- Emergency treatment of hyperkalaemia (p. 260)

Administration
- Hyperglycaemia

  Soluble insulin (e.g. Actrapid) 50 units made up to 50 ml with sodium chloride 0.9%
  Adjust rate according to the sliding scale below

Insulin sliding scale:

Blood sugar (mmol/l)	Rate (ml/h)
<3.5	0
3.6–5.5	1
5.6–7.0	2
7.1–9.0	3
9.1–11.0	4
11.1–17.0	5
>17.0	6

The energy and carbohydrate intake must be adequate; this may be in the form of enteral or parenteral feeding, or IV infusion of glucose 10% containing 10–40 mmol/l KCl running at a constant rate appropriate to the patient's fluid requirements (85–125 ml/h). The blood glucose concentration should be maintained between 4 and 10 mmol/l

Monitor:
Blood glucose 2 hourly until stable then 4 hourly
Serum potassium 12 hourly

How not to use insulin
SC administration not recommended for fine control. Adsorption of insulin occurs with PVC bags (use polypropylene syringes). If an insulin infusion is running with feed and that feed is interrupted, e.g. for the patient to go for a scan, then the insulin rate should be reduced and re-titrated. This is a common cause of hypoglycaemia

Adverse effects
Hypoglycaemia

Cautions
Insulin resistance may occur in patients with high levels of IgG antibodies to insulin, obesity, acanthosis nigricans and insulin receptor defects. Co-administration of corticosteroids and inotropes may adversely affect glycaemic control

IPRATROPIUM

An antimuscarinic bronchodilator traditionally regarded as more effective in relieving bronchoconstriction associated with COPD.

Uses
Reverse bronchospasm, particularly in COPD

Administration
- Nebuliser: 250–500 µg up to 6 hourly, undiluted (if prolonged delivery time desirable then dilute with sodium chloride 0.9% only)
- For patients with chronic bronchitis and hypercapnia, oxygen in high concentration can be dangerous, and nebulisers should be driven by air

How not to use ipratropium
For nebuliser: do not dilute in anything other than sodium chloride 0.9% (hypotonic solution may cause bronchospasm). Ipratropium is not a logical choice for patients with thick secretions as ipratropium may make these worse

Adverse effects
Dry mouth
Tachycardia
Paradoxical bronchospasm (stop giving if suspected)
Acute angle closure glaucoma (avoid escape from mask to patient's eyes)

Cautions
Prostatic hypertrophy – urinary retention (unless patient's bladder catheterised)

ISOPRENALINE

Isoprenaline is a β_1- and β_2-adrenoceptor agonist causing: ↑ HR, ↑ automaticity, ↑ contractility, ↓ diastolic BP, ↑ systolic BP, ↑ myocardial oxygen demand and bronchodilation. It has a half-life of <5 min.

Uses
Complete heart block, while getting temporary pacing established

Contraindications
Tachyarrhythmias
Heart block caused by digoxin

Administration
- IV infusion: up to 20 μg/min

  4 mg made up to 50 ml glucose 5% (80 μg/ml)

Dose (μg/min)	Infusion rate (ml/h)
1	0.75
2	1.5
4	3
10	7.5
20	15

How not to use isoprenaline
Do not use sodium chloride 0.9% as a diluent

Adverse effects
Tachycardia
Arrhythmias
Angina
Hypotension

Cautions
Risk of arrhythmias with concurrent use of other sympathomimetics and volatile anaesthetics

KETAMINE (Ketalar)

Ketamine is a non-competitive antagonist of N-methyl-D-aspartate (NMDA) receptors and also binds to *mu* and *kappa* opioid receptors. It is licensed as an anaesthetic agent for diagnostic and surgical procedures and is best suited to shorter procedures. It has a role in the ICU as a co-analgesic, with opioid-sparing properties. It has good analgesic properties in subanaesthetic doses. Use of midazolam or another benzodiazepine as an adjunct to ketamine reduces the incidence of emergence reactions.

Ketamine has also been used for treatment of patients with severe asthma, as it has bronchodilating properties probably deriving from two different mechanisms – firstly, via a central effect inducing catecholamine release, thereby stimulating β2 adrenergic receptors, and secondly, by inhibition of vagal pathways to produce an anticholinergic effect acting directly on bronchial smooth muscle. Ketamine is metabolised in the liver to an active metabolite – norketamine. This has a potency of around one-third that of ketamine. The metabolites are then excreted renally with an elimination half-life of 2–3 hours in adults. Orally administered ketamine undergoes extensive first-pass metabolism in the liver, resulting in a bioavailability of ~16%.

Ketamine is used recreationally and is illicitly obtained from healthcare sources. Ketamine exerts strong hallucinogenic and euphoric effects, and it is often combined with other club drugs, where it is snorted, injected or ingested. In the UK, ketamine is classified as a 'controlled drug' (CD), and many hospitals require full CD governance (although this is not required by law). Overuse can cause catatonia, inducing a dissociative state, users describe as falling into a 'k-hole'. Ketamine-induced ulcerative cystitis, 'ketamine bladder' can occur with 'ketamine addicts' or 'near-daily' users.

Uses

As a co-analgesic with opioids (unlicensed), for bronchodilation in asthma (unlicensed)
Anaesthetic for short procedures and intubation

Contraindications

Where elevation of blood pressure would constitute a serious hazard
Eclampsia or pre-eclampsia
Severe coronary or myocardial disease
Cerebrovascular accident or cerebral trauma

How not to use ketamine

Ketamine should not be mixed in the same syringe/bag as barbiturates or diazepam as a precipitate will form

Administration

All doses are expressed as the base: 1.15 mg ketamine hydrochloride 1 mg of base

- Analgesia: IV infusion: 10–45 mcg/kg/min adjusted according to response, alternatively IV loading dose 2–3 mg/kg, can be followed by IV infusion: 5–10 mg/hour or IM: 1.5–2 mg/kg
- Anaesthesia: IM short procedures: initially 6.5–13 mg/kg (10 mg/kg usually gives 12–25 minutes of surgical anaesthesia); painful diagnostic manoeuvres: initially 4 mg/kg IV
- Intubation: 1–2 mg/kg IV over 2–4 minutes
- Oral ketamine (unlicensed route), e.g. for dressing changes, the IV preparation can be given orally 6 mg/kg; this takes 20 mins to take effect. This dose causes hypersalivation in 20% of cases. May be administered with glycopyrrollate (to counteract hypersalivation) and midazolam (to counteract hallucination)

Ketamine is available as 200 mg/20 ml, 500 mg/10 ml and 1,000 mg/10 ml vials. The 200 mg/20 ml and 500 mg/10 ml solutions may be used undiluted. The 1,000 mg/10 ml vial should be diluted with an equal volume of sodium chloride 0.9% or glucose 5% to produce a 50 mg/ml solution

Adverse effects

Jaundice
Tachycardia
Hypertension
Delirium
Lowering the seizure threshold
Hallucination
Hypersalivation
Nausea, vomiting
Dizziness and headache

Cautions

Mild-to-moderate hypertension and tachyarrhythmia
Chronic alcoholism and acute alcohol intoxication
Elevated cerebrospinal fluid pressure
Globe injuries and increased intraocular pressure
Neurotic traits or psychiatric illness (e.g. schizophrenia and acute psychosis)
Acute intermittent porphyria
Seizures
Hyperthyroidism or patients receiving thyroid replacement (increased risk of hypertension and tachycardia)
Pulmonary or upper respiratory tract infection (ketamine sensitises the gag reflex, potentially causing laryngospasm)
Intracranial mass lesions, a presence of head injury, or hydrocephalus
Daily use for a few weeks can cause dependence and tolerance
Ketamine and theophylline reduces the seizure threshold

Ketamine may potentiate the neuromuscular blocking effects of atracurium
Ketamine antagonises the hypnotic effect of thiopental
With antihypertensives – enhanced hypotensive effect

Organ failure
Renal: no dose adjustment needed
Liver: mild–moderate hepatic cirrhosis, use usual initial dose then halve subsequent doses
Severe hepatic cirrhosis – no information available – manufacturer advises use only if potential benefit outweighs risk

K

LABETALOL (Trandate)

Labetalol is a combined α- and β-adrenoceptor antagonist. The proportion of β-blockade to α-blockade when given orally is 3:1, and 7:1 when given IV. It lowers the blood pressure by blocking α-adrenoceptors in arterioles and thereby reduces the peripheral resistance. Concurrent β-blockade protects the heart from reflex sympathetic drive normally induced by peripheral vasodilatation.

Uses
All grades of hypertension, particularly useful when there is tachycardia
Pre-eclampsia

Contraindications
Asthma (worsens)
Cardiogenic shock (further myocardial depression)
Second- or third-degree heart block

Administration
- Orally: 100–800 mg 12 hourly
- IV bolus: 10–20 mg over 2 min, repeat with 40 mg at 10-min intervals as necessary, up to 300 mg in 24 hours

  Maximum effect usually occurs within 5 min and the duration of action is usually 6 hours

- IV infusion: 20–200 mg/h

  Rate: 4–40 ml/h (20–200 mg/h), adjust rate until satisfactory decrease in BP obtained
  Available in 20-ml ampoules containing 100 mg labetalol (5 mg/ml)
  Draw up three ampoules (60 ml) into a 50-ml syringe

How not to use labetalol
Incompatible with sodium bicarbonate

Adverse effects
Postural hypotension
Bradycardia
Heart failure

Cautions
Rare reports of severe hepatocellular damage (usually reversible)
Presence of labetalol metabolites in urine may result in false-positive test for phaeochromocytoma

Organ failure
Hepatic: reduce dose

LACTULOSE

L

Lactulose is a semi-synthetic disaccharide that is not absorbed from the GI tract. It produces an osmotic diarrhoea of low faecal pH, and discourages the proliferation of ammonia-producing organisms.

Uses
Constipation
Hepatic encephalopathy

Contraindications
Intestinal obstruction
Galactosaemia

Administration
• Constipation

   Orally: 15 ml 12 hourly, gradually reduced according to patient's needs
   May take up to 48 h to act

• Hepatic encephalopathy

   Orally: 30–50 ml 8 hourly, subsequently adjusted to produce 2–3 soft stools daily

Adverse effects
Flatulence
Abdominal discomfort

LACTULOSE

LEVETIRACETAM (Keppra)

The use of this broad-spectrum anti-epileptic is expanding in the acute setting. It can be given via a number of routes as it is available in IV, tablet and liquid formulations. Monitoring of levels is unnecessary, which simplifies therapy compared with phenytoin and phenobarbital. It is better tolerated than carbamazepine and has few interactions.

Uses
It is licensed for monotherapy and adjunctive treatment of focal sei zures with or without secondary generalisation, and for adjunctive therapy of myoclonic seizures in patients with juvenile myoclonic epilepsy and primary generalised tonic-clonic seizures; although experi-ence is accumulating in nonconvulsive status epilepticus (if not responding to phenytoin/phenobarbital).

Contraindications
Hypersensitivity to levetiracetam or excipients

Administration
- A gradual increase in dose is recommended to minimise cognitive side effects as follows: initially 500 mg twice daily increased after 1–2 weeks by 1 g daily until anti-epileptic control is achieved; max. 1.5 g twice daily. However, in the ICU, experience suggests that this can be speeded up (unlicensed) in an acute scenario with an initial dose of 1 g bd

  When switching between IV and oral routes of administration, the dose is the same, as absorption is nearly 100%

  IV: add the dose to 100 ml of sodium chloride 0.9% or glucose 5% and administer over 15 minutes. Each 500 mg vial contains 2.5 mmol sodium

How not to use levetiracetam (Keppra)
Do not withdraw chronic therapy abruptly

Adverse effects
Hypotension, headache, somnolence
Depression, aggression, anxiety, insomnia, irritability
Eucopenia, neutropenia, pancytopenia, alopecia, toxic epidermal necrolysis, Stevens–Johnson syndrome
Anorexia, cough, asthenia/fatigue

Cautions
Withdraw established therapy slowly, e.g. 500 mg decreases twice daily every 2–4 weeks to avoid precipitating an increase in the frequency of seizures.

Organ failure

Renal: max. 2 g daily if CC 50–80 ml/min; max. 1.5 g daily if CC 30–50 ml/min; max. 1 g daily if CC less than 30 ml/min

Liver: halve dose in severe hepatic impairment if CC < 60 ml/min

Renal replacement therapy

Dosing dependent on clearance rate as described in Short Notes Renal Replacement Therapy (p. 300–303)

L

LEVETIRACETAM (Keppra)

LEVOSIMENDAN

Levosimendan is licensed in several countries for the treatment of acute decompensated congestive heart failure (CHF). Levosimendan acts by sensitizing the myocardium to calcium so that a greater ventricular contraction (cardiac output) can be achieved without increasing oxygen requirements. Levosimendan also causes coronary and systemic vasodilation, mediated by activation of ATP-sensitive sarcolemmal K-channels, and activation of ATP-sensitive mitochondrial K-channels. Levosimendan has also been shown to possess anti-inflammatory properties. As part of the systemic inflammatory response, myocardial dysfunction is commonly associated with severe sepsis. The calcium sensitising and anti-inflammatory actions of levosimendan provide a strong rationale for its use in sepsis. Studies have shown that levosimendan increases cardiac output and lowers cardiac filling pressures and is associated with a reduction of cardiac symptoms, risk of death and hospitalisation. Its action is independent of interactions with β-adrenergic receptors. Noradrenaline is the initial vasopressor of choice. Vasopressin may be added in resistant hypotension. It is important to use the lowest dose of vasopressor to achieve an acceptable MAP to allow tissue perfusion. Additional inotropic agents may be required. Dobutamine, adrenaline and milrinone may be used in the presence of low cardiac output after fluid resuscitation. Levosimendan has a short plasma half-life of approximately 1 hour, is around 95% bound to plasma proteins and is fully metabolised in the liver and intestine into both active and inactive metabolites. Although the infusion is for 24 hours only, the haemodynamic effects persist for up to 7 days, due to the effects of the active metabolite, OR-1896.

Uses
Acute decompensation of severe chronic heart failure despite maximal standard therapy
Low cardiac output syndrome or cardiogenic shock
Septic shock refractory to inotropes (unlicensed)

Contraindications
Right heart failure
High-output failure
Congenital heart disease
Isolated diastolic dysfunction
Hypertrophic cardiomyopathy
Uncorrected stenotic valve disease
Endocarditis

Administration
- Supplied as 5 ml ampoules containing 12.5 mg levosimendan in 2.5 mg/ml
- Withdraw 5 ml from a 500 ml bag of glucose 5% and replace with 5 ml (12.5 mg) levosimendan

- Final concentration of infusion is 25 µg/ml. Administer peripherally or centrally
- No loading dose required. Start with continuous infusion of 0.1 µg/kg/min and if tolerated after 2–4 hours increase to 0.2 µg/kg/min for a duration of 24 hours in total. In the event of excessive hypotension or tachycardia, reduce rate to 0.05 µg/kg/min.

Dosage (ml/h):

Weight (kg)	Infusion rate at 0.1 µg/kg/min (ml/h)	Infusion rate at 0.2 µg/kg/min (ml/h)	Infusion rate at 0.05 µg/kg/min (ml/h)
40	10	19	5
50	12	24	6
60	14	29	7
70	17	34	8
80	19	38	10
90	22	43	11
100	24	48	12
110	26	53	13
120	29	58	14
130	31	62	16

Adverse effects
Headache
Hypotension (<15%)
Arrhythmias (<10%)
Myocardial ischaemia

Cautions
Hypotension (exacerbation)
Use with milronone or enoximone as levosimendan may also have phosphodiesterase inhibitory effects
Hepatic failure (reduced clearance)

Organ failure
Renal: unknown, but in practice the dose is not adjusted. Active metabolite (ORG 1896) is renally cleared and has a long half-life of ~80 hours

L

LIDOCAINE

This anti-arrhythmic agent suppresses automaticity of conduction and spontaneous depolarisation of the ventricles during diastole. Clearance is related to both hepatic blood flow and hepatic function; it will be prolonged in liver disease, cardiac failure and the elderly. The effects after the initial bolus dose last about 20 min. An IV infusion is needed to maintain the anti-arrhythmic effect.

Uses
Prevention of ventricular ectopic beats, VT and VF after MI

Contraindications
It is no longer the first-line drug in pulseless VT or VF during cardiac arrest
Hypersensitivity to amide-type local anaesthetics (rare)
Heart block (risk of asystole)

Administration
- Loading dose:
  1.5 mg/kg IV over 2 min, repeat after 5 min to a total dose of 3 mg/kg if necessary. Reduce dose in the elderly

- Maintenance dose:
  4 mg/min for 1st hour
  2 mg/min for 2nd hour
  1 mg/min thereafter

Reduce infusion rates in patients with hepatic impairment, cardiac failure and in the elderly
  Undiluted 40 ml 2% solution (800 mg)
  4 mg/min = 12 ml/h
  2 mg/min = 6 ml/h
  1 mg/min = 3 ml/h

Continuous ECG and BP monitoring

How not to use lidocaine
Do not give by rapid IV bolus (should not be given at >50 mg/min)

Adverse effects
Paraesthesia, muscle twitching, tinnitus
Anxiety, drowsiness, confusion, convulsions
Hypotension, bradycardia, asystole

Cautions
Elderly (reduced volume of distribution, reduce dose by 50%)
Hepatic impairment
Cardiac failure
Other class 1 anti-arrhythmics, e.g. phenytoin, may increase risk of toxicity

Organ failure
Cardiac: reduce dose
Hepatic: reduce dose

LINEZOLID (Zyvox)

The first example of a new class of antibiotics called the oxazolidinones. It is a reversible, non-selective MAOI. It is highly effective against all Gram +ve organisms including MRSA, penicillin-resistant pneumococci and VRE (vancomycin-resistant enterococci). Emergence of resistance during therapy has been uncommon to date. Linezolid is a useful alternative to the glycopeptides (teicoplanin and vancomycin) in patients with renal impairment as it is not known to be nephrotoxic, and does not require therapeutic dosage monitoring. The oral route (tablets or suspension) has good bioavailability and is therefore given at the same dose as the IV formulation.

Uses
Community-acquired pneumonia
Nosocomial pneumonia (combined with antibiotic active against Gram −ve organisms)
Severe infections due to MRSA
Complicated skin and soft tissue infections
Infections due to VRE

Contraindications
Concurrent use of MAOIs (Types A or B) or within 2 weeks of taking such drugs

Administration
Recommended duration of treatment is 10–14 consecutive days. Safety and effectiveness of linezolid when administered for periods longer than 28 days have not been established

Oral: 600 mg 12 hourly
Also available as suspension (100 mg/5 ml) 30 ml 12 hourly
IV: 600 mg (300-ml bag containing 2 mg/ml solution) 12 hourly infused over 30–120 min

Monitor FBC weekly (risk of reversible myelosuppression)

How not to use linezolid
Currently licensed for up to 14 days therapy only (risk of myelosuppression may increase with longer duration)

Adverse effects
Oral and vaginal candidiasis
Diarrhoea
Nausea
Reversible myelosuppression
Headaches

Cautions

Severe renal failure

Unless close BP monitoring possible, avoid in uncontrolled hypertension, phaeochromocytoma, carcinoid tumour, thyrotoxicosis and patients on SSRIs, tricyclic antidepressants, pethidine, buspirone or sympathomimetics or dopaminergic drugs

Organ failure

Renal: no dose adjustment required
Hepatic: no dose adjustment required

LIOTHYRONINE

Liothyronine has a similar action to levothyroxine but has a more rapid effect and is more rapidly metabolised. Its effects develop after a few hours and disappear within 1–2 days of discontinuing treatment. It is available both as a tablet for oral administration and as a solution for slow intravenous injection. It is useful in severe hypothyroid states when a rapid response is desired. If adverse effects occur due to excessive dosage, withhold for 1–2 days and restart at a lower dose. The injectable form is useful in patients unable to absorb enterally.

Uses
Replacement for those unable to absorb enterally
Hypothyroid states, including coma

Contraindications
Thyrotoxicosis

Administration
Hypothyroid coma: 5–20 μg (neat or diluted in 5 ml WFI), given by slow IV over 5 min, 12 hourly. Give concurrent hydrocortisone 100 mg IV, 8 hourly, especially if pituitary hypothyroidism suspected

Replacement for those unable to absorb enterally: 5–20 μg (neat or diluted in 5 ml WFI), given by slow IV over 5 min, 12 hourly, depending on the normal dose of levothyroxine

Equivalent dose:

Oral levothyroxine (μg/day)	IV liothyronine (μg/12 h)
200	20
150	15
100	10
50	5

Monitor:
ECG before and during treatment
TSH (T3 and T4 may be unreliable in the critically ill)
Normal range: TSH 0.5–5.7 mU/l, T3 1.2–3.0 nmol/l, T4 70–140 nmol/l

How not to use liothyronine
Rapid IV bolus

L

Adverse effects
Tachycardia
Arrhythmias
Angina
Muscle cramps
Restlessness
Tremors

Cautions
Panhypopituitarism or predisposition to adrenal insufficiency (give hydrocortisone before liothyronine)
IHD (may worsen ischaemia)

LOPERAMIDE

L

Reduces GI motility by direct effect on nerve endings and intramural ganglia within the intestinal wall. Very little is absorbed systemically.

Uses
Acute or chronic diarrhoea

Contraindications
Bowel obstruction
Toxic megacolon
Pseudomembranous colitis

Administration
Orally: 4 mg, then 2 mg after each loose stool to a usual maximum of 16 mg/day
To reduce high output from stoma, doses of up to 30 mg four times daily have been used (unlicensed dose) – liquid not suitable for this indication, tablets are preferable
Available in 2 mg capsules/tablets and 1 mg/5 ml syrup
Stools should be cultured

Adverse effects
Bloating
Abdominal pain

LORAZEPAM (Ativan)

Lorazepam may now be the preferred first-line drug for stopping status epilepticus (p. 272). Although it may have a slower onset of action, it carries a lower risk of cardiorespiratory depression (respiratory arrest, hypotension) than diazepam as it is less lipid soluble. Lorazepam also has a longer duration of anticonvulsant activity compared with diazepam (6–12 hours versus 15–30 min after a single bolus).

Uses
Termination of epileptic fit

Contraindications
Airway obstruction

Administration
- IV: 4 mg over 2 min, repeated after 10 min if no response
- IM: 4 mg, dilute with 1 ml of WFI or sodium chloride 0.9%

Ampoules stored in refrigerator between 0°C and 4°C

How not to use lorazepam
IM injection – painful and unpredictable absorption; only use when IV route not possible

Adverse effects
Respiratory depression and apnoea
Drowsiness
Hypotension and bradycardia

Cautions
Airway obstruction with further neurological damage
Enhanced and prolonged sedative effect in the elderly
Additive effects with other CNS depressants

Organ failure
CNS: enhanced and prolonged sedative effect
Respiratory: ↑ respiratory depression
Hepatic: enhanced and prolonged sedative effect. Can precipitate coma
Renal: enhanced and prolonged sedative effect

MAGNESIUM SULPHATE

Like potassium, magnesium is one of the major cations of the body responsible for neurotransmission and neuromuscular excitability. Regulation of magnesium balance is mainly by the kidneys.

Hypomagnesaemia may result from failure to supply adequate intake, from excess NG drainage or suctioning or in acute pancreatitis. It is usually accompanied by a loss of potassium. The patient may become confused and irritable, with muscle twitching.

Hypomagnesaemia should also be suspected in association with other fluid and electrolyte disturbances when the patient develops unexpected neurological features or cardiac arrhythmias.

Magnesium sulphate has long been the mainstay of treatment for preeclampsia/eclampsia in America, but the practice in the UK until recently has been to use more specific anti-convulsant and antihypertensive agents. A large international collaborative trial shows a lower risk of recurrent convulsions in eclamptic mothers given magnesium sulphate compared with those given diazepam or phenytoin.

Normal serum magnesium concentration: 0.7–1.0 mmol/l

Therapeutic range for pre-eclampsia/eclampsia: 2.0–3.5 mmol/l

Uses
Hypomagnesaemia
Hypomagnesaemia associated with cardiac arrhythmias
Pre-eclampsia
Anticonvulsant in eclampsia
Acute asthma attack
Cardiac arrest (p. 257)

Contraindications
Hypocalcaemia (further $\downarrow Ca^{2+}$)
Heart block (risk of arrhythmias)
Oliguria

Administration

Magnesium sulphate solution for injection

Concentration (%)	g/ml	mEq/ml	mmol/ml
10	0.1	0.8	0.4
25	0.25	2	1
50	0.5	4	2

1 g = 8 mEq = 4 mmol

- Hypomagnesaemia

  IV infusion: 10 mmol magnesium sulphate made up to 50 ml with glucose 5%
  Do not give at >30 mmol/h
  Repeat until plasma level is normal
  Concentrations <20% are suitable for peripheral IV administration

- Hypomagnesaemia associated with cardiac arrhythmias

  IV infusion: 20 mmol diluted in 100 ml glucose 5%, given over 1 h
  Do not give at >30 mmol/h
  Repeat until plasma level is normal
  Concentrations <20% are suitable for peripheral IV administration

- Pre-eclampsia/eclampsia

  Loading dose: 4 g (8 ml 50% solution) diluted in 250 ml sodium chloride 0.9% IV, given over 10 min
  Maintenance: 1 g/h IV, as necessary. Add 10 ml 50% magnesium sulphate to 40 ml sodium chloride 0.9% and infuse at 10 ml/h
  Newborn – monitor for hyporeflexia and respiratory depression

- Acute asthma: 2 g in 50 ml sodium chloride 0.9% IV, given over 20 min

Oral therapy

- Magnesium glycero phosphate (unlicensed product) 1 g tablets contain 4 mmol of Mg^{2+}. Usual starting adult dose 1–2 tablets 8 hourly

Monitor: BP
        respiratory rate
        ECG
        tendon reflexes
        renal function
        serum magnesium level

Maintain urine output >30 ml/h

How not to use magnesium sulphate

Rapid IV infusion can cause respiratory or cardiac arrest
IM injections (risk of abscess formation)

Adverse effects

Related to serum level:

- 4.0–6.5 mmol/l

    Nausea and vomiting
    Somnolence
    Double vision
    Slurred speech
    Loss of patellar reflex

- 6.5–7.5 mmol/l

    Muscle weakness and paralysis
    Respiratory arrest
    Bradycardia, arrhythmias and hypotension

- >10 mmol/l

    Cardiac arrest

Plasma concentrations >4.0 mmol/l cause toxicity which may be treated with calcium gluconate 1 g IV (10 ml 10%)

Cautions

- Oliguria and renal impairment (↑ risk of toxic levels)
- Potentiates both depolarising and non–depolarising muscle relaxants

Organ failure

Renal: reduce dose and slower infusion rate, closer monitoring for signs of toxicity

Renal replacement therapy

Removed by CVVH/HF/PD. Accumulates in renal failure, monitor levels

M

MAGNESIUM SULPHATE

MANNITOL

An alcohol capable of causing an osmotic diuresis. Available as 10% and 20% solutions. Crystallisation may occur at low temperatures. It has a rapid onset of action and duration of action is up to 4 h. Rapid infusion of mannitol increases the cardiac output and the BP.

Uses
Cerebral oedema
Preserve renal function peri–operatively in jaundiced patients
To initiate diuresis in transplanted kidneys
Rhabdomyolysis

Contraindications
Congestive cardiac failure
Pulmonary oedema (acute expansion of blood volume)
↑ Intravascular volume (further ↑ intravascular volume)

Administration
- Cerebral oedema

   IV infusion: 0.5–1.0 g/kg as a 20% solution, given over 30 min

Weight (kg)	Volume of 20% mannitol at 0.5 g/kg (ml)
60	150
70	175
80	200
90	225
100	250

100 ml 20% solution = 20 g

- Jaundice

Pre–operative:
   Insert urinary catheter
   1000 ml sodium choride 0.9% over 1 h, 2 h before surgery
   250 ml 20% mannitol over 30 min, 1 h before surgery

Peri–operative:
   200–500 ml 20% mannitol if urine output <60 ml/h
   sodium chloride 0.9% to match urine output

- Kidney transplant

   IV infusion: 0.5–1.0 g/kg over 30 min, given with furosemide 40 mg
   IV on reperfusion of transplanted kidney

- Rhabdomyolysis

IV infusion: 0.5–1.0 g/kg as a 20% solution over 30–60 min

M

How not to use mannitol
Do not give in the same line as blood
Only give mannitol to reduce ICP when the cause is likely to be relieved surgically (rebound increase in ICP)

Adverse effects
Fluid overload
Hyponatraemia and hypokalaemia
Rebound ↑ ICP

Cautions
Extravasation (thrombophlebitis)

Organ failure
Cardiac: worsens
Renal: fluid overload

Renal replacement therapy
No further dose modification is required during renal replacement therapy

MEROPENEM (Meronem)

Meropenem is similar to imipenem but is stable to the renal enzyme dehydropeptidase–1, which inactivates imipenem. Meropenem is also less likely to induce seizures than imipenem. Meropenem has an extremely wide spectrum of activity, including most aerobic and anaerobic Gram −ve and +ve bacteria (but not MRSA).

Uses
Meningitis
Mixed aerobic/anaerobic infections
Presumptive therapy of a wide range of severe infections prior to availability of sensitivities
Febrile neutropenia

Contraindications
Hypersensitivity to beta lactams
Infections caused by MRSA

Administration

- IV: 0.5–1 g 8 hourly, given over 5 min

  Reconstitute with 10 ml WFI

- IV infusion: 0.5–1 g 8 hourly, give over 15–30 min

  For meningitis, increase to 2 g 8 hourly

In renal impairment:
Monitor:

CC (ml/min)	Dose*	Interval (h)
20–50	1 unit dose	12
10–20	0.5 unit dose	12
<10	0.5 unit dose	24

*Based on unit doses of 0.5, 1 or 2 g

FBC
LFT

Adverse effects
Thrombophlebitis
Hypersensitivity reactions
Positive Coombs' test
Reversible thrombocythaemia, thrombocytopenia, eosinophilia and neutropenia
Abnormal LFT (↑ bilirubin, transaminases and alkaline phosphatase)

Cautions
Hypersensitivity to penicillins and cephalosporins
Hepatic impairment
Renal impairment
Concurrent use of nephrotoxic drugs

Organ failure
Hepatic: worsens
Renal: reduce dose

Renal replacement therapy
CVVH dialysed, dependent on clearance rate as described in Short Notes
Renal Replacement Therapy (p. 300–303) and CC table given previously.
HD/PD dialysed, dose as in CC <10 ml/min i.e. 500 mg–1 g every
24 hours

METARAMINOL (Aramine)

Uses
Hypotension (for patients without central venous access)

Contraindications
Peripheral or mesenteric vascular thrombosis (may extend infraction area)
Profound hypoxia or hypercapnia (risk of arrhythmias)

Administration
• IV bolus: 0.5–1 mg, given over 3 min

Reconstitute with 10 ml WFI

• IV infusion: 0.5–5 mg/h

Titrate the infusion rate according to the patient's BP
Draw up two ampoules of metaraminol (10 mg in 1 ml) in a 60 ml syringe. Make up to 40 ml with sodium chloride 0.9% or glucose 5%. The concentration of the final solution is 20 mg in 40 ml (0.5 mg/ml)

Adverse effects
Hypertension
Bradycardia
Arrhythmias

Cautions
Extravasation (phentolamine may be beneficial)

METHYLPREDNISOLONE

Methylprednisolone is a potent corticosteroid with anti-inflammatory activity at least five times that of hydrocortisone. It has greater gluco-corticoid activity and insignificant mineralocorticoid activity, making it particularly suitable for conditions where sodium and water retention would be a disadvantage. Corticosteroids have been suggested to reduce lung inflammation in ARDS. The fibroproliferative phase occurs between 7 and 14 days from the onset of ARDS. There are no large controlled trials at present to show conclusive benefit from this practice.

Uses
Fibroproliferative phase of ARDS (unlicensed)

Adjunct in *Pneumocystis carinii* pneumonia (see co-trimoxazole and pentamidine)

Contraindications
Systemic infection (unless specific anti-microbial therapy given)

Administration
- Fibroproliferative phase of ARDS (unlicensed)

  IV infusion: 2 mg/kg loading dose (rounded to nearest 20 mg) then 0.5 mg/kg (rounded to the nearest 10 mg) 6 hourly for 14 days or until extubation whichever is quicker. Then convert to prednisolone 1 mg/kg orally each morning for 7 days, then 0.5 mg/kg each morning for 7 days daily, then 0.25 mg/kg for 2 days, then 0.125 mg/kg for 2 days then stop

- Adjunct in *Pneumocystis carinii* pneumonia (see co-trimoxazole and pentamidine)

  IV infusion: 1 g once daily for 3 days; if the patient responds well steroids may be stopped, if not continue as follows: days 4 and 5 500 mg IV once daily, then days 6–16 prednisolone reducing regimen, i.e. 60 mg, 50 mg, 40 mg, 30 mg, 20 mg 15 mg, 10 mg, 10 mg, 5 mg, 5 mg then stop

The steroid should be started at the same time as the co-trimoxazole or pentamidine and should be withdrawn before the antibiotic treatment is complete

Reconstitute with WFI. Make up to 50 ml sodium chloride 0.9% or glucose 5% give over at least 30 min

How not to use methylprednisolone
Do not give by rapid IV injection (hypotension, arrhythmia, cardiac arrest)

Avoid live virus vaccinations

Adverse effects

Prolonged use may also lead to the following problems:

- increased susceptibility to infections
- impaired wound healing
- peptic ulceration
- muscle weakness (proximal myopathy)
- osteoporosis
- hyperglycaemia

Cautions

Diabetes mellitus
Concurrent use of NSAID (increased risk of GI bleeding)

METOCLOPRAMIDE

Metoclopramide acts by promoting gastric emptying, increasing gut motility and has an anti-emetic effect. It raises the threshold of the chemoreceptor trigger zone. In high doses it has $5\text{-}HT_3$ antagonist action.

Uses
Anti-emetic
Promotes gastric emptying
Increases lower oesophageal sphincter tone

Administration
• IV/IM/PO/NG: 10 mg 8 hourly

How not to use metoclopramide
Orally not appropriate if actively vomiting
Rapid IV bolus (hypotension)

Adverse effects
Extrapyramidal movements
Neuroleptic malignant syndrome

Cautions
Increased risk of extrapyramidal side-effects occurs in the following:

• hepatic and renal impairment
• children, young adults (especially girls) and the very old
• concurrent use of anti-psychotics
• concurrent use of lithium

Treatment of acute oculogyric crises includes stopping metoclopramide (usually subside within 24 hours) or giving procyclidine 5–10 mg IV (usually effective within 5 min)

Organ failure
Hepatic: reduce dose
Renal: reduce dose

Renal replacement therapy
No further dose modification is required during renal replacement therapy

METOPROLOL

Metoprolol is a selective β_1-adrenoreceptor blocking agent; this prefer-
ential effect is not absolute, however, and at higher doses it also inhibits
β_2-adrenoreceptors. Plasma levels following oral administration are
approximately 50% of levels following IV administration, indicating
about 50% first-pass metabolism. For dose conversion purposes, equivalent maximal beta-blocking effect is achieved with oral and IV doses
in the ratio of approximately 2.5:1. Metoprolol is eliminated mainly by
bio-transformation in the liver, and the plasma half-life ranges from
approximately 3 to 7 hours. Hence, no reduction in dosage is usually
needed in patients with renal failure.

Uses
Hypertension
Angina pectoris
Control of tachyarrhythmias
Myocardial infarction

Contraindications
Asthma (worsens unless compelling reasons for use)
Second- or third-degree heart block
Decompensated cardiac failure (pulmonary oedema, hypoperfusion or
hypotension)

Administration
    Orally: usually 25–50 mg 8–12 hourly
    IV bolus: initially up to 5 mg at a rate of 1–2 mg/min; can be
    repeated at 5-min intervals until a satisfactory response. A total dose
    of 10–15 mg generally proves sufficient
    IV infusion (unlicensed): dilute 20 mg in 50 ml of sodium chloride
    0.9% or glucose 5%. Starting dose 0.04 mg/kg/h and titrate to
    response, usually up to 0.1 mg/kg/h

Adverse effects
Bradycardia
Heart failure
Postural hypotension

Cautions
Subject to enzyme inducers and inhibitors (p. 248)
Increased negative inotropic and chronotropic effects may occur when
metoprolol is given with verapamil and diltiazem. Avoid IV verapamil
in patients treated with beta-blockers

Organ failure
Hepatic: reduce dose

METRONIDAZOLE

High activity against anaerobic bacteria and protozoa. It is also effective in the treatment of *Clostridium difficile*-associated disease preferably given by the oral route. IV metronidazole may be used in patients with impaired gastric emptying and/or ileus.

Uses
Clostridium difficile-associated diarrhoea
Anaerobic infections
Protozoal infections (*Trichomonas vaginalis*, *Giardia intestinalis* and amoebic dysentery)
Bacterial vaginosis
Eradication of *Helicobacter pylori*

Administration
* *Clostridium difficile*-associated diarrhoea

  Orally: 400 mg 8 hourly
  IV: 500 mg 8 hourly

* Anaerobic infections

  IV: 500 mg 8 hourly
  PR: 1 g 8 hourly

* Eradication of *Helicobacter pylori*

Metronidazole 400 mg PO/NG 12 hourly and proton pump inhibitor standard dose (e.g. lansoprazole 30 mg/omeprazole 20 mg) PO/NG 12 hourly and amoxicillin 1 g PO/NG 12 hourly or clarithromycin 500 mg PO/NG 12 hourly; all for 7 days. IV eradication therapy has less evidence of success than oral; therefore preferably wait until PO/NG route is available

Adverse effects
Nausea and vomiting
Unpleasant taste
Rashes, urticaria and angioedema
Darkening of urine
Peripheral neuropathy (prolonged treatment)

Cautions
Hepatic impairment
Disulfiram-like reaction with alcohol

MICAFUNGIN (Mycamine)

Micafungin (Mycamine) is an echinocandin, similar to caspofungin and anidulafungin. It covers a wide range of *Candida* species causing invasive candidiasis, including *C. krusei* and *C. glabrata*. The key distinguishing features compared with caspofungin are simplicity of dosing regimen (no loading dose), storage at room temperature, narrower clinical indication and fewer drug interactions.

Uses
Invasive candidiasis
Oesophageal candidiasis
Prophylaxis of *Candida* infection in neutropenic patients

Contraindications
Hypersensitivity to echinocandin

Administration
- Invasive candidiasis

  IV infusion: 100 mg once daily, given over 1 hour (increase to 200 mg daily if inadequate response) for a minimum of 14 days
  Weight < 40 kg, 2 mg/kg once daily, given over 1 hour (increase to 4 mg/kg daily if inadequate response)

- Oesophageal candidiasis

  IV infusion: 150 mg once daily, given over 1 hour for at least one week after resolution of infection
  Weight < 40 kg, 3 mg/kg once daily, given over 1 hour

- Prophylaxis of *Candida* infection in neutropenic patients

  IV infusion: 50 mg once daily, given over 1 hour for at least one week after neutrophil recovery
  Weight < 40 kg, 1 mg/kg once daily, given over 1 hour

Reconstitute each vial with 5 ml sodium chloride 0.9% or glucose 5%. Gently rotate vial, without shaking. Add the reconstituted solution to 100 ml sodium chloride 0.9% or glucose 5%. Protect from light. Available in vials containing 50 mg and 100 mg

How not to use micafungin
Galactose intolerance
Severe hepatic failure

M

Adverse effects
Headaches
Diarrhoea, nausea and vomiting
Leukopenia, neutropenia, anaemia and thrombocytopenia
Increased creatinine
Hypokalaemia, hypomagnesaemia and hypocalcaemia
Elevated LFTs
Flushing
Rash
Pruritus

Cautions
Hepatic failure (worsening LFTs)
Breast feeding and pregnancy

Organ failure
Renal: no dose adjustment necessary, as negligible renal clearance
Hepatic: avoid in severe liver failure

Renal replacement therapy
Unlikely to be removed by dialysis, therefore no dose adjustment required

MICAFUNGIN (Mycamine)

MIDAZOLAM

Midazolam is a water-soluble benzodiazepine with a short duration of action (elimination half-life 1–4 hours). However, prolonged coma has been reported in some critically ill patients usually after prolonged infusions. Midazolam is metabolised to the metabolite α-hydroxy midazolam, which is rapidly conjugated. Accumulation of midazolam after prolonged sedation has been observed in critically ill patients. In renal failure the glucuronide may also accumulate, causing narcosis.

Uses
Sedation
Anxiolysis

Contraindications
As an analgesic
Airway obstruction

Administration
- IV bolus: 2.5–5 mg PRN
- IV infusion: 0.5–6 mg/h

Administer neat or diluted in glucose 5% or sodium chloride 0.9%
Titrate dose to level of sedation required

Stop or reduce infusion each day until patient awakes, when it is restarted. Failure to assess daily will result in delayed awakening when infusion is finally stopped

Time to end effects after infusion: 30 min to 2 hours (but see below).

How not to use midazolam
The use of flumazenil after prolonged use may produce confusion, toxic psychosis, convulsions, or a condition resembling delirium tremens

Adverse effects
Residual and prolonged sedation
Respiratory depression and apnoea
Hypotension

M

Cautions
Enhanced and prolonged sedative effect results from interaction with:

- opioid analgesics
- antidepressants
- antihistamines
- α–blockers
- anti–psychotics

Enhanced effect in the elderly and in patients with hypovolaemia, vasoconstriction or hypothermia

Midazolam is metabolised by the hepatic microsomal enzyme system (cytochrome P450s). Induction of the P450 enzyme system by another drug can gradually increase the rate of metabolism of midazolam, resulting in lower plasma concentrations and a reduced effect. Conversely inhibition of the metabolism of midazolam results in a higher plasma concentration and an increased effect. Examples of enzyme inducers and inhibitors are listed on p. 248

Flumazenil is a specific, but short–acting, antagonist (p. 101)

Organ failure
CNS: sedative effects increased
Cardiac: exaggerated hypotension
Respiratory: ↑ respiratory depression
Hepatic: enhanced and prolonged sedative effect. Can precipitate coma
Renal: increased cerebral sensitivity

Renal replacement therapy
No further dose modification is required during renal replacement therapy, although accumulation of active metabolite will occur in renal failure so care is required to avoid prolonged sedation upon cessation of midazolam

MIDAZOLAM

MILRINONE

Milrinone is a selective phosphodiesterase III inhibitor resulting in ↑ CO, and ↓ PCWP and SVR, without significant ↑ in HR and myocardial oxygen consumption. It produces slight enhancement in AV node conduction and may ↑ ventricular rate in uncontrolled AF/atrial flutter.

Uses
Severe congestive cardiac failure

Contraindications
Severe aortic or pulmonary stenosis (exaggerated hypotension)
Hypertrophic obstructive cardiomyopathy (exaggerated hypotension)

Administration
• IV infusion: 50 μg/kg loading dose over 10 min, then maintain on 0.375–0.75 μg/kg/min to a maximum haemodynamic effect

Requires direct arterial BP monitoring
Adjustment of the infusion rate should be made according to haemodynamic response
Available in 10-ml ampoules containing 10 mg milrinone (1 mg/ml)
Dilute this 10 ml solution with 40 ml sodium chloride 0.9% or glucose 5% giving a solution containing milrinone 200 μg/ml

Dose (μg/kg/min)	Infusion rate (ml/kg/h)
0.375	0.11
0.4	0.12
0.5	0.15
0.6	0.18
0.7	0.21
0.75	0.22

Maximum daily dose: 1.13 mg/kg

In renal impairment:

CC (ml/min)	Dose (μg/kg/min)
20–50	0.28–0.43
<10–20	0.23–0.28
<10	0.2–0.23

How not to use milrinone
Furosemide and bumetanide should not be given in the same line as milrinone (precipitation)

Adverse effects
Hypotension
Arrhythmias

Cautions
Uncontrolled AF/atrial flutter

Organ failure
Renal: reduce dose

Renal replacement therapy
No further dose modification is required during renal replacement therapy

MORPHINE

Morphine is the standard opioid with which others are compared and remains a valuable drug for the treatment of acute, severe pain. Peak effect after IV bolus is 15 min. Duration of action is between 2 and 3 hours. Both liver and kidney function are responsible for morphine elimination. The liver mainly metabolises it. One of the principal metabolites, morphine 6-glucuronide (M6G), is also a potent opioid agonist and may accumulate in renal failure.

Uses
Relief of severe pain
To facilitate mechanical ventilation
Acute left ventricular failure — by relieving anxiety and producing vasodilatation

Contraindications
Airway obstruction
Pain caused by biliary colic

Administration
- IV bolus: 2.5 mg every 15 min PRN
- IV infusion rate: 1–5 mg/h

  Dilute in glucose 5% or sodium chloride 0.9%
  Stop or reduce infusion each day and restart when first signs of discomfort appear. Failure to assess daily will result in overdosage and difficulty in weaning patient from ventilation

- If the patient is conscious the best method is to give an infusion pump they can control (PCA): 50 mg made up to 50 ml with sodium chloride 0.9%; IV bolus: 1 mg; lockout: 3–10 min

How not to use morphine
In combination with an opioid partial agonist, e.g. buprenorphine (antagonises opioid effects)

Adverse effects
Respiratory depression and apnoea
Hypotension and tachycardia
Nausea and vomiting
Delayed gastric emptying
Reduced intestinal mobility
Biliary spasm
Constipation
Urinary retention
Histamine release
Tolerance
Pulmonary oedema

Cautions

Enhanced and prolonged effect when used in patients with renal failure, the elderly and in patients with hypovolaemia and hypothermia. Enhanced sedative and respiratory depression from interaction with:

- benzodiazepines
- antidepressants
- anti-psychotics

Head injury and neurosurgical patients (may exacerbate $\uparrow$ ICP as a result of $\uparrow$ PaCO$_2$)

Organ failure

CNS: sedative effects increased
Respiratory: $\uparrow$ respiratory depression
Hepatic: can precipitate coma
Renal: increased cerebral sensitivity. M6G accumulates

Renal replacement therapy

CVVH dialysed dependent on clearance rate as described in Short Notes Renal Replacement Therapy (p. 300–303), typically use a smaller dose than usual, e.g. 2.5–5 mg. HD dialysed dose as in CC <10 ml/min, i.e. use smaller doses, e.g. 1.25–2.5 mg and extended dosing intervals. PD not dialysable, dose as per HD. Active metabolite M6G accumulates in renal failure. Titrate to response, such as pain/sedation scores

M

NALOXONE

This is a specific opioid antagonist. The elimination half-life is 60–90 min, with a duration of action between 30 and 45 min.

Uses
Reversal of opioid adverse effects – respiratory depression, sedation, pruritus and urinary retention
As a diagnostic test of opioid overdose in an unconscious patient

Contraindications
Patients physically dependent on opioids

Administration
- Reversal of opioid overdose: 200 μg IV bolus, repeat every 2–3 min until desired response, up to a total of 2 mg
- Infusion may be required in patients with renal impairment or those who had taken long-acting opioids, e.g. MST, usual starting dose is 60% of initial IV bolus dose infused over 1 hour, then adjusted according to respiratory rate and level of consciousness, e.g. if the initial bolus is 1 mg, the infusion is started at 0.6 mg/hour. Dilute 10 mg to 50 ml with sodium chloride 0.9% or glucose 5%
- Reversal of spinal opioid-induced pruritus: dilute 200 μg in 10 ml WFI. Give 20 μg boluses every 5 min until symptoms resolve

Titrate dose carefully in postoperative patients to avoid sudden return of severe pain

How not to use naloxone
Large doses should not be given quickly

Adverse effects
Arrhythmias
Hypertension

Cautions
Withdrawal reactions in patients on long-term opioid for medical reasons or in addicts
Postoperative patients – return of pain and severe haemodynamic disturbances (hypertension, VT/VF, pulmonary oedema)

Organ failure
Hepatic: delayed elimination

NEOSTIGMINE

N

Neostigmine is a cholinesterase inhibitor leading to prolongation of ACh action. This will enhance parasympathetic activity in the gut and increase intestinal motility. When used for acute colonic pseudo–obstruction, organic obstruction of the gut must first be excluded and it should not be used shortly after bowel anastomosis (Ponec RJ, et al. *N Engl J Med* 1999; **341**: 137–41). Colonic pseudo–obstruction, which is the massive dilation of the colon in the absence of mechanical obstruction, can develop after surgery or severe illness. Most cases respond to conservative treatment. In patients who do not respond, colonic decompression is often performed to prevent ischaemia and perforation of the bowel. Colonoscopy in these patients is not always successful and can be accompanied by complications such as perforation.

Uses
Colonic pseudo–obstruction (unlicensed)

Administration
- IV bolus: 2.5 mg, repeated 3 hours later if no response to initial dose
  Monitor ECG (may need to give atropine or other anticholinergic drugs to counteract symptomatic bradycardia)

Contraindications
Mechanical bowel obstruction
Urinary obstruction

How not to use neostigmine
It should not be used shortly after bowel anastomosis

Adverse effects
Increased sweating
Excess salivation
Nausea and vomiting
Abdominal cramp
Diarrhoea
Bradycardia
Hypotension
These muscarinic side-effects are antagonised by atropine

Cautions
Asthma

Organ failure
Renal: reduce dose

Renal replacement therapy
No further dose modification is required during renal replacement therapy

NIMODIPINE

A calcium–channel blocker with smooth muscle relaxant effect preferentially in the cerebral arteries. Its use is confined to prevention of vascular spasm after subarachnoid haemorrhage. Nimodipine is used in conjunction with the 'triple H' regimen of hypertension, hypervolaemia and haemodilution to a haematocrit of 30–33.

Uses
Subarachnoid haemorrhage

Administration
- IV infusion

  1 mg/h, ↑ to 2 mg/h if BP not severely ↓
  If <70 kg or BP unstable start at 0.5 mg/h
  Ready prepared solution – do not dilute, but administer into a running infusion (40 ml/h) of sodium chloride 0.9% or glucose 5%, via a central line
  Continue for between 5 and 14 days
  Use only polyethylene or polypropylene infusion sets
  Protect from light

  10 mg in 50 ml vial (0.02%)
  0.5 mg/h = 2.5 ml/h
  1 mg/h = 5 ml/h
  2 mg/h = 10 ml/h

- Orally (prophylaxis)

  60 mg every 4 hours for 21 days

How not to use nimodipine
Avoid PVC infusion sets
Do not use peripheral venous access
Do not give nimodipine tablets and IV infusion concurrently
Avoid concurrent use of other calcium-channel blockers, β-blockers or nephrotoxic drugs

Adverse effects
Hypotension (vasodilatation)
Transient ↑ liver enzymes with IV use

Cautions
Hypotension (may be counterproductive by ↓ cerebral perfusion)
Cerebral oedema or severely ↑ ICP
Renal impairment

NORADRENALINE

The α_1 effect predominates over its β_1 effect, raising the BP by increasing the SVR. It increases the myocardial oxygen requirement without increasing coronary blood flow. Noradrenaline (norepinephrine) reduces renal, hepatic and muscle blood flow, but in septic shock, noradrenaline may increase renal blood flow and enhance urine production by increasing perfusion pressure. Acute renal failure secondary to inadequate renal perfusion is a common form of kidney failure seen in the ICU. Once intravascular volume has been restored, the MAP should be restored to a level that optimally preserves renal perfusion pressure i.e. above 65 mmHg (or higher in previously hypertensive patients).

Uses
Septic shock, with low SVR

Contraindications
Hypovolaemic shock
Acute myocardial ischaemia or MI

Administration
• Usual dose range: 0.01–0.4 µg/kg/min IV infusion via a central vein

Initially start at a higher rate than intended, to increase the BP more rapidly, and then reduce rate
4 mg made up to 50 ml glucose 5% (80 µg/ml)

Dosage chart (ml/h):

Weight (kg)	Dose (µg/kg/min)				
	0.02	0.05	0.1	0.15	0.2
50	0.8	1.9	3.8	5.6	7.5
60	0.9	2.3	4.5	6.8	9
70	1.1	2.6	5.3	7.9	10.5
80	1.2	3	6	9	12
90	1.4	3.4	6.8	10.1	13.5
100	1.5	3.8	7.5	11.3	15
110	1.7	4.1	8.3	12.4	16.5
120	1.8	4.5	9	13.5	18

How not to use noradrenaline

In the absence of haemodynamic monitoring

Do not use a peripheral vein (risk of extravasation)

Do not connect to CVP lumen used for monitoring pressure (surge of drug during flushing of line)

Adverse effects

Bradycardia

Hypertension

Arrhythmias

Myocardial ischaemia

Cautions

Hypertension

Heart disease

If extravasation of noradrenaline occurs – phentolamine 10 mg in 15 ml sodium chloride 0.9% should be infiltrated into the ischaemic area with a 23-G needle

NYSTATIN

Nystatin is a polyene antifungal which is not absorbed when given orally and is too toxic for IV use.

Uses
Oral candida infection
Suppression of gut carriage of candida
Topical therapy of genital candida infections

Administration
• Oral candidiasis

  1 ml (100 000 units) 6 hourly, holding in mouth

How not to use nystatin
IV too toxic

Adverse effects
Rash
Oral irritation

OCTREOTIDE

Octreotide is an analogue of somatostatin. It is used to provide relief from symptoms associated with carcinoid tumours and acromegaly. It may also be used for the prevention of complications following pancreatic surgery. For patients undergoing pancreatic surgery, the peri- and postoperative administration of octreotide reduces the incidence of typical postoperative complications (e.g. pancreatic fistula, abscess and subsequent sepsis, postoperative acute pancreatitis). Octreotide exerts an inhibiting effect on gallbladder motility, bile acid secretion and bile flow, and there is an acknowledged association with the development of gallstones in prolonged usage.

Uses
Prevention of complications following pancreatic surgery
Pancreatic leak (unlicensed)
Variceal haemorrhage (2nd line to terlipressin)

Administration
- Prevention of complications following pancreatic surgery

  SC or IV: 100 µg 8 hourly for 7 days, starting on the day of operation at least one hour before laparotomy

- Pancreatic leak

SC or IV: 100–200 µg 8 hourly
To reduce pain and irritation on injection, allow solution to reach room temperature and rotate injection site
IV dose should be diluted with 5 ml sodium chloride 0.9%
Available as 50, 100 and 500 µg/1 ml ampoules. Use the 500 µg/1 ml ampoule for SC injection of doses ≥200 µg to reduce pain arising from the injection volume
Variceal haemorrhage (unlicensed indication): only use if terlipressin is contraindicated (e.g. ischaemic ECG). Dose 100 µg IV stat then a continuous infusion of 50 µg/h continued for 24 hours after variceal banding. Then reduce dose to 25 µg/h for 12 hours then stop. To prepare solution dilute 5 × 100 µg ampoules to 50 ml with sodium chloride 0.9% = 10 µg/ml solution. 50 µg/h = 5 ml/h; 25 µg/h = 2.5 ml/h
Dilute to a ratio of not less than 1:1 and not more than 1:9 by volume

Stored in fridge at 2–8°C

How not to use octreotide
Abrupt withdrawal (biliary colic and pancreatitis)
Dilution with solution containing glucose is not recommended

Adverse effects

GI disturbances (nausea, vomiting, pain, bloating and diarrhoea)

Pain and irritation at injection site (allow solution to reach room temperature and rotate injection sites)

Elevated LFTs

Gallstone formation with prolonged use

Cautions

Growth hormone-secreting pituitary tumour (may increase in size)

Insulinoma (hypoglycaemia)

Requirement for insulin and oral hypoglycaemic drugs may be reduced in diabetes mellitus

Organ failure

Hepatic: reduce dose

OCTREOTIDE

OLANZAPINE (Zyprexa)

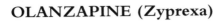

This is an atypical antipsychotic agent that is a dopamine D_1, D_2, D_4, 5-HT_2, histamine-1 and muscarinic-receptor antagonist.

Although licensed for conditions such as acute schizophrenia and mania, there is emerging literature (*Intensive Care Med* 2004; **30**: 444–9) of using this agent as an alternative to haloperidol in delirium. It also offers an alternative parenteral (IM) option for management of acute agitation. For NG therapy, there is a dispersible tablet, which will also dissolve on the tongue.

Uses
Management of delirium in ICU patients (unlicensed), especially in prolonged QT interval as an alternative to benzodiazepines. Licensed indications: schizophrenia, mania, either alone or as combination therapy, preventing recurrence in bipolar disorder. The IM preparation is used for control of agitation and disturbed behaviour in schizophrenia or mania.

Contraindications
Patients with known risk for narrow-angle glaucoma

Administration
Delirium PO/NG 5 mg daily (elderly 2.5 mg daily); adjusted to usual range of 5–20 mg daily; max. 20 mg daily

Control of agitation, IM initially 5–10 mg (usual dose 10 mg) then 5–10 mg after 2 hours if needed. Elderly initially 2.5–5 mg as a single dose followed by 2.5–5 mg after 2 hours if necessary. Max. 3 injections daily for 3 days. Max. daily combined oral and parenteral dose 20 mg

Available as 5, 10, 15 and 20 mg tabs and dispersible tabs; IM 10 mg

How not to use IM olanzapine
IM injections are not suitable for thrombocytopenic patients, as risk of bleeding

Adverse effects
Transient antimuscarinic effects
Drowsiness, speech difficulty, hallucinations, fatigue
Increased temperature, oedema plus eosinophilia
Less commonly hypotension, bradycardia, QT-interval prolongation, seizures, leucopenia and rash
IM: sinus pause and hypoventilation

Cautions
QT prolongation
Increased risk of hypotension, bradycardia and respiratory depression when IM olanzapine given with IV benzodiazepines

Increased risk of side effects including neutropenia when olanzapine given with valproate

Increased risk of ventricular arrhythmias with anti-arrhythmics that prolong the QT interval

Increase plasma concentration of tricyclics, possibly increased risk of ventricular arrhythmias

Antagonise anticonvulsant effect of antiepileptics (convulsive threshold lowered)

Organ failure

Renal: consider initial dose 5 mg
Liver: consider initial dose 5 mg

OLANZAPINE (Zyprexa)

OMEPRAZOLE

Omeprazole is a proton pump inhibitor (PPI) which inhibits gastric acid production by the gastric parietal cells. Following endoscopic treatment of bleeding peptic ulcers, omeprazole given intravenouly for 72 hours has been shown to reduce the risk of rebleeding (*N Engl J Med* 2000; **343**: 310–6). PPIs are often overused in the ICU and there is emerging data linking PPI use with *Clostridium difficile* infection (Dial S, *et al*. *CMAJ* 2004; **171**: 33–8).

Uses
Bleeding peptic ulcers, after endoscopic treatment of bleeding (unlicensed)
Continuation of PPI therapy when the PO/NG route is unavailable
Helicobacter pylori eradication

Administration
- Bleeding peptic ulcers, after endoscopic treatment of bleeding

  IV: Initial 80 mg IV loading dose given over 1 hour, followed by 8 mg/h
  IV infusion for 72 hours
  Reconstitute with either sodium chloride 0.9% or glucose 5%
  See appendix G

- Continuation of PPI therapy when the PO/NG route is unavailable

  IV bolus: 40 mg daily. Reconstitute 40 mg vial with the solvent provided and administer over 5 min

- Eradication of *Helicobacter pylori*

  See monograph on metronidazole

Adverse effects
GI disturbances (nausea, vomiting, abdominal pain, diarrhoea and constipation)
Paraesthesia
Agitation
Liver dysfunction
Hyponatraemia
Leukopenia and thrombocytopenia rarely

Cautions
Severe hepatic disease (risk of encephalopathy)
Pregnancy (toxic in animal studies)
May mask symptoms of gastric cancer
Omeprazole may enhance anticoagulant effect of warfarin – monitor INR and may increase phenytoin levels
Omeprazole may reduce the effectiveness of clopidogrel

Organ failure
Hepatic: reduce dose

ONDANSETRON

A specific 5-HT$_3$ antagonist. Its efficacy is enhanced by addition of dexamethasone.

Uses
Severe post–operative nausea and vomiting (PONV)
Highly emetogenic chemotherapy

Administration
- PONV

    IV bolus: 4 mg over 3–5 min when required up to 8 hourly. Dose may be doubled

- Highly emetogenic chemotherapy

    IV bolus: 8 mg over 3–5 min, followed by two doses of 8 mg 2–4 hourly or continuous IV infusion of 1 mg/h for up to 24 hours

Dilution: 24 mg ondansetron made up to 48 ml with sodium chloride 0.9% or glucose 5%
Rate of infusion: 2 ml/h

How not to use ondansetron
Do not give rapidly as IV bolus

Adverse effects
Headaches
Flushing
Constipation
Increases in liver enzymes (transient)

Cautions
Hepatic impairment

Organ failure
Hepatic: reduced clearance (moderate or severe liver disease: not > 8 mg daily)

PABRINEX IVHP (INTRAVENOUS HIGH POTENCY)

Wernicke's encephalopathy can be difficult to diagnose, and the consequences of leaving it untreated can be devastating. Pabrinex is a combination of water-soluble vitamins B and C, which is used parenterally to rapidly treat severe depletion or malabsorption, particularly after alcoholism. As thiamine does not exist as a licensed parenteral product, Pabrinex is widely used to treat and prevent Wernicke's encephalopathy. An alternative approach is to use an unlicensed IV thiamine product. Pabrinex IVHP is supplied in two ampoules which contain:

Ampoule no. 1 (5 ml)
Thiamine hydrochloride (Vit B_1) 250 mg
Riboflavin (Vit B_2) 4 mg
Pyridoxine hydrochloride (Vit B_6) 50 mg

Ampoule no. 2 (5 ml)
Ascorbic acid (Vit C) 500 mg
Nicotinamide (Vit B_3) 160 mg
Anhydrous glucose 1000 mg

Note: a double-strength ampoule pair exists of 10 ml. All doses mentioned here refer to the 5 ml product.

Uses
Treatment and prevention of Wernicke's encephalopathy

At-risk groups: Alcohol misusers
Eating disorders
Long-term parenteral nutrition
Hyperemesis gravidarum
Dialysis

Lactic acidosis secondary to beriberi

Administration
To prepare Pabrinex IVHP: draw up contents of both ampoules numbers 1 and 2 into one syringe and mix. Add this to 50–100 ml of sodium chloride 0.9% and administer over 30 min

Pabrinex should be administered before parenteral glucose is given, as in thiamine deficiency IV glucose may worsen symptoms and increase thiamine requirements

Prevention of Wernicke's encephalopathy: one pair of IVHP 5-ml ampoules once or twice daily for 3–5 days

Treatment of Wernicke's encephalopathy or beriberi: Two pairs of IVHP 5-ml ampoules 8 hourly for 3 days. If no response is seen, discontinue therapy; if a response is seen, decrease the dose to one pair of ampoules daily for as long as improvement continues. When the Pabrinex course is finished, give oral thiamine 50–100 mg 8 hourly and 1–2 multivitamin tablets daily for the rest of admission. For severe vitamin B group deficiency, give 1–2 vitamin B compound strong tablets 8 hourly. A short course of folic acid may also be beneficial

How not to give Pabrinex
Do not confuse the IV product with the IM preparation, nor the 5 and 10 ml product

Adverse effects
Occasional hypotension and mild paraesthesia

Cautions
Anaphylactic shock rarely

PANCURONIUM

A non-depolarising neuromuscular blocker with a long duration of action (1–2 h). It is largely excreted unchanged by the kidneys. It causes a 20% increase in HR and BP. It may be a suitable choice in the hypotensive patient, although the tachycardia induced may not be desirable if the HR is already high, e.g. hypovolaemia, septic shock.

Uses
Patients where prolonged muscle relaxation is desirable, e.g. intractable status asthmaticus

Contraindications
Airway obstruction
To facilitate tracheal intubation in patients at risk of regurgitation
Renal and hepatic failure (prolonged paralysis)
Severe muscle atrophy
Tetanus (sympathomimetic effects)

Administration
- Initial dose: 50–100 µg/kg IV bolus
- Incremental doses: 20 µg/kg, every 1–2 h

Monitor with peripheral nerve stimulator

How not to use pancuronium
As part of a rapid sequence induction
In the conscious patient
By persons not trained to intubate trachea

Adverse effects
Tachycardia and hypertension
Prolonged use (disuse muscle atrophy)

Cautions
Breathing circuit (disconnection)
Prolonged use (disuse muscle atrophy)

Organ failure
Hepatic: prolonged paralysis
Renal: prolonged paralysis

Renal replacement therapy
No further dose modification is required during renal replacement therapy

PANTOPRAZOLE

Pantoprazole is a proton pump inhibitor (PPI), similar to omeprazole. The injectable formulation can be used as an alternative to omeprazole. PPIs are often overused in the ICU and there are emerging data linking PPI use with *Clostridium difficile* infection (Dial S, et al. *CMAJ* 2004; **171**: 33–8).

Uses
Bleeding peptic ulcers, after endoscopic treatment of bleeding (unlicensed)
Continuation of PPI therapy when the PO/NG route is unavailable
Helicobacter pylori eradication

Administration
• Bleeding peptic ulcers, after endoscopic treatment of bleeding

IV: Initial 80 mg IV loading dose given over 1 hour, followed by 8 mg/h IV infusion for 72 hours
Reconstitute with either sodium chloride 0.9% or glucose 5%

• Continuation of PPI therapy when the PO/NG route is unavailable

IV: 40 mg daily. Reconstitute 40 mg vial with the 10 ml sodium chloride 0.9%; administer as a slow bolus. Alternatively, add to 100-ml bag of sodium chloride 0.9% or glucose 5% and administer over 15 min or as a continuous infusion (unlicensed).

Adverse effects
GI disturbances (abdominal pain, diarrhoea, flatulence and constipation)
Headache
Agitation
Liver dysfunction
Leukopenia and thrombocytopenia rarely

Cautions
Severe hepatic disease (risk of encephalopathy)
Pregnancy (toxic in animal studies)
May mask symptoms of gastric cancer
Pantoprazole may enhance anticoagulant effect of warfarin – monitor INR
Pantoprazole may reduce the effectiveness of clopidogrel

Organ failure
Hepatic: reduce 40 mg dose to 20 mg
Renal: no dose adjustment is necessary

P

PARACETAMOL

The efficacy of single-dose IV paracetamol as a post-operative analgesic has been confirmed by many studies. The IV formulation provides a more predictable plasma concentration and has potency slightly less than that of a standard dose of morphine or the NSAIDs. The mechanism of action remains unclear as, unlike opioids and NSAIDs respectively, paracetamol has no known endogenous binding sites and does not inhibit peripheral cyclooxygenase activity significantly. There is increasing evidence of a central antinociceptive effect, and potential mechanisms for this include inhibition of a central nervous system COX-2, inhibition of a putative central cyclooxygenase 'COX-3' that is selectively susceptible to paracetamol, and modulation of inhibitory descending serotinergic pathways. Paracetamol has also been shown to prevent prostaglandin production at the cellular transcriptional level, independent of cyclooxygenase activity.

The availability of intravenous paracetamol (Perfalgan) will enhance and extend the use of this drug as a fundamental component of multimodal analgesia after surgery and in critically ill patients who are not able to absorb enterally. The dose differs between IV and oral paracetamol (oral bioavailability is around 75%–95% relative to IV dose). An average adult could safely be given up to 4 g oral paracetamol daily and 4 g IV.

Uses
Mild to moderate pain
Fever

Administration
Oral or PR: 0.5–1 g every 4–6 hours; maximum of 4 g daily
IV infusion: 1 g (100 ml) given over 15 min, every 4–6 hours; max. 4 g daily,
>50 kg with additional risk factors for hepatotoxicity, max. 3 g daily,
<50 kg, 15 mg/kg up to 6 hourly

How not to use paracetamol
Do not exceed 4 g/day
Do not use the standard IV dose for patients weighing below 50 kg

Adverse effects
Hypotension with IV infusion
Liver damage with overdose

Cautions
Hepatic impairment
Renal impairment
Alcohol dependence

Organ failure
Hepatic: avoid large doses (dose-related toxicity)
Renal: increase IV infusion dose interval to every 8 hours if creatinine
    clearance <10 ml/min

P

PARACETAMOL

PENTAMIDINE

Pentamidine isetionate given by the intravenous route is an alternative for patients with severe *Pneumocystis carinii* (now renamed *Pneumocystis jirovecii*) pneumonia unable to tolerate co-trimoxazole, or who have not responded to it. Pentamidine isetionate is a toxic drug and personnel handling the drug must be adequately protected. Nebulised pentamidine may be used for mild disease and for prophylaxis. Thin-walled air-containing cysts (pneumatoceles) and pneumathoraces are more common in patients receiving nebulised pentamidine as prophylaxis. Adverse effects, sometimes severe, are more common with pentamidine than co-trimoxazole.

Uses
Alternative treatment for severe *Pneumocystis carinii* pneumonia (PCP)

Administration
- IV infusion: 4 mg/kg every 24 hours for at least 14 days

  Dilute in 250 ml glucose 5%, given over 1–2 hours

In renal impairment:

CC (ml/min)	Dose (mg/kg)	Interval (h)
10–50	4	24
<10	4	24 for 7–10 days then on alternate days to complete a minimum of 14 doses

Adjuvant corticosteroid has been shown to improve survival. The steroid should be started at the same time as the pentamidine and should be withdrawn before the antibiotic treatment is complete. Oral prednisolone 50–80 mg daily or IV hydrocortisone 100 mg 6 hourly or IV dexamethasone 8 mg 6 hourly or IV methylprednisolone 1 g for 5 days, then dose reduced to complete 21 days of treatment

How not to use pentamidine
Nebulised route not recommended in severe PCP ($\downarrow$ PaO$_2$)
Concurrent use of both co-trimoxazole and pentamidine is not of benefit and may increase the incidence of serious side-effects

Adverse effects
Acute renal failure (usually isolated $\uparrow$ serum creatinine)
Leucopenia, thrombocytopenia
Severe hypotension
Hypoglycaemia
Pancreatitis
Arrhythmias

P

Cautions
Blood disorders
Hypotension
Renal/hepatic impairment

Organ failure
Renal: reduce dose

Renal replacement therapy
No further dose modification is required during renal replacement
therapy

PENTAMIDINE

P

PETHIDINE

Pethidine has one-tenth the analgesic potency of morphine. The duration of action is between 2 and 4 h. It has atropine-like actions and relaxes smooth muscles. The principal metabolite is norpethidine, which can cause fits. In renal failure and after infusions this metabolite can accumulate and cause seizures.

Uses
It may be indicated in controlling pain from pancreatitis, secondary to gallstones, and after surgical procedure involving bowel anastomosis, where it is claimed to cause less increase in intraluminal pressure

It produces less release of histamine than morphine, and may be preferable in asthmatics

Contraindications
Airway obstruction
Concomitant use of MAOI

Administration
*   IV bolus: 10–50 mg PRN

    Duration of action: 2–3 hours

*   PCAS: 600 mg in 60 ml sodium chloride 0.9%

    IV bolus: 10 mg, lockout 5–10 min

How not to use pethidine
In combination with an opioid partial agonist, e.g. buprenorphine (antagonises opioid effects)

Adverse effects
Respiratory depression and apnoea
Hypotension and tachycardia
Nausea and vomiting
Delayed gastric emptying
Reduce intestinal mobility
Constipation
Urinary retention
Histamine release
Tolerance
Pulmonary oedema

Cautions
Enhanced sedative and respiratory depression from interaction with:

*   benzodiazepines
*   antidepressants
*   anti-psychotics

P

Avoid concomitant use of and for 2 weeks after MAOI discontinued (risk of CNS excitation or depression – hypertension, hyperpyrexia, convulsions and coma)

Head injury and neurosurgical patients (may exacerbate ↑ ICP as a result of ↑ PaCO$_2$)

Organ failure
CNS: sedative effects increased
Respiratory: ↑ respiratory depression
Hepatic: enhanced and prolonged sedative effect. Can precipitate coma
Renal: increased cerebral sensitivity. Norpethidine accumulates

Renal replacement therapy
No further dose modification is required during renal replacement therapy

PHENOBARBITAL SODIUM (PHENOBARBITONE)

The bioavailability of phenobarbital is 90%, so the IV dose can be regarded as the same as the oral dose. With a half-life of 1.4–4.9 days, steady-state may take 5–14 days to be reached. Therapeutic serum levels for seizures range from 10 to 40 mg/l although the optimal plasma concentration for some individuals may vary outside this range. Phenobarbital usually lowers phenytoin levels but they can also be increased. Laboratory levels may be reported in μmol/l or mg/l. To convert mg/l into μmol/l multiply by 4.31.

Uses
Status epilepticus (p. 270)

Contraindications
Porphyria

Administration
- IV: 10 mg/kg (maximum daily dose 1 g)

  Dilute to 10 times its own volume with WFI immediately before use. Give at <100 mg/min

Phenobarbital can be continued at a rate of 50 mg/min until seizures cease; maximum cumulative dose in the absence of intubation, 20 mg/kg. Reduce dose and inject more slowly in the elderly, patients with severe hepatic and renal impairment, and in hypovolaemic and shocked patients. Maintenance dose: 1 mg/kg IV 12 hourly (average maintenance dose 30–60 mg 12 hourly). To discontinue therapy, wean off slowly over several weeks by reducing daily dose by 15–30 mg/day every fortnight. In obese patients, dosage should be based on lean body mass

Adverse effects
Respiratory depression
Hypotension
Bradycardia
CNS depression

Organ failure
CNS: sedative effects increased
Respiratory: ↑ respiratory depression
Hepatic: can precipitate coma
Renal: reduce dose

Renal replacement therapy
No further dose modification is required during renal replacement therapy

PHENTOLAMINE

Phentolamine is a short-acting α-blocker that produces peripheral vasodilatation by blocking both α_1- and α_2-adrenergic receptors. Pulmonary vascular resistance and pulmonary arterial pressure are decreased.

Uses
Severe hypertension associated with phaeochromocytoma

Contraindications
Hypotension

Administration
Available in 10-mg ampoules

- IV bolus: 2–5 mg, repeat PRN
- IV infusion: 0.1–2 mg/min

Dilute in sodium chloride 0.9% or glucose 5%
Monitor pulse and BP continuously

How not to use phentolamine
Do not use adrenaline, ephedrine, isoprenaline or dobutamine to treat phentolamine-induced hypotension (β_2 effect of these sympathomimetics will predominate causing a further paradoxical $\downarrow$ BP)

Treat phentolamine-induced hypotension with noradrenaline

Adverse effects
Hypotension
Tachycardia and arrhythmias
Dizziness
Nasal congestion

Cautions
Asthma (sulphites in ampoule may lead to hypersensitivity)
IHD

P

PHENYTOIN

Phenytoin is approximately 90% protein bound. Plasma levels are based on total phenytoin (bound plus free) and dosage must be adjusted when serum albumin is reduced (see equation below). Hypoalbuminaemia will lead to an increased fraction of unbound drug. The free fraction is responsible for the pharmacological action of the drug. Phenytoin demonstrates zero-order kinetics and does not demonstrate a proportional relationship between drug levels and dose. Maintenance dosage should not be increased by increments of more than 50–100 mg per day.

Uses
Status epilepticus (p. 270)
Anticonvulsant prophylaxis in post-neurosurgical operations
Anti-arrhythmic – particularly for arrhythmias associated with digoxin toxicity

Contraindications
Do not use IV phenytoin in sino-atrial block, or second- and third-degree AV block

Administration
- Status epilepticus:

  IV bolus: 20 mg/kg (max. 2 g) dilute in 100–250 ml sodium chloride 0.9%, given at a rate ≤50 mg/min
  IV infusion: 100 mg diluted in 50–100 ml sodium chloride 0.9%, given over 30–60 min, 8 hourly for maintenance
  Give through a 0.2 micron filter, via large vein or central vein
  Available in 5 ml ampoules containing 250 mg phenytoin

- Anticonvulsant prophylaxis:

  PO/IV: 200–600 mg/day

- Anti-arrhythmic:

  IV: 100 mg every 15 min until arrhythmia stops. Maximum 15 mg/kg/day

Monitor:

  ECG and BP
  Serum phenytoin level (p. 250)
Recommended therapeutic range 40–80 μmol/l or 10–20 mg/l

Hypoalbuminaemia will lead to an increased fraction of unbound active drug. The reported total phenytoin (bound + free) levels are open to misinterpretation because an apparently 'normal' level in a hypoalbuminaemic patient may hide a toxic level of free phenytoin. A conceptual corrected level can be determined, which reflects what the total phenytoin level would be if the patient had normal protein levels. To adjust for a low albumin:

Adjusted phenytoin level = reported level ÷ [(0.02 × serum albumin) + 0.1]

PHENYTOIN

However, this equation depends on the accurate measurement of serum albumin. Some albumin assays are not reliable below 15 g/l. If available, free phenytoin levels are preferable if the albumin is low

If the patient is fitting and levels are low:

• Consider a loading dose:

Loading dose (mg) = 0.67 × weight (kg) × change in plasma concentration required (in mg/l)

• Increase maintenance dose as follows:

<7 mg/l level, increase daily dose by 100 mg daily
7–12 mg/l level, increase daily dose by 50 mg daily
12–16 mg/l level, increase daily dose by 25 mg daily

NG administration and IV to oral/NG conversion: theoretically one should take account of the different salts of the IV and liquid preparation but in practice one can use a 1-to-1 conversion, but give the oral/NG as a single daily dose. Note that enteral feed reduces the absorption of phenytoin liquid so stop feed for 2 hours before and 2 hours after phenytoin administration. In practice, conversion from IV to NG phenytoin at the same total daily dose often results in reduced levels

How not to use phenytoin
Rapid IV bolus not recommended (hypotension, arrhythmias, CNS depression)
Do not dissolve in solutions containing glucose (precipitation)
IM injection not recommended (absorption slow and erratic)
Do not give into an artery (gangrene)
Do not prescribe NG phenytoin three times daily, as feed will be turned off for 9 hours per day

Adverse effects
Nystagmus, ataxia and slurred speech
Drowsiness and confusion
Hypotension (rapid IV)
Prolonged QT interval and arrhythmias (rapid IV)
Gingival hyperplasia (long-term)
Rashes
Aplastic anaemia
Agranulocytosis
Folate deficiency
Megaloblastic anaemia
Thrombocytopenia

Cautions
Severe liver disease (reduce dose)
Metabolism subject to other enzyme inducers and inhibitors (p. 248)
Additive CNS depression with other CNS depressants

Organ failure
CNS: enhanced sedation
Hepatic: increased serum level

P

PHOSPHATES

Hypophosphataemia may lead to muscle weakness and is a cause of difficulty in weaning a patient from mechanical ventilation. Causes of hypophosphataemia in ICU include failure of supplementation (e.g. during TPN), malnutrition, diarrhoea, use of insulin and high concentration glucose, continuous renal replacement therapy and use of loop diuretics. Intravenous therapy is generally recommended in symptomatic hypophosphataemia and phosphate levels <0.32 mmol/l. Hypophosphataemia may lead to a multitude of symptoms, including cardiac and respiratory failure, and is associated with higher mortality although it is unknown if correction of hypophosphataemia improves mortality (Geerse et al., *Critical Care* 2010; **14**: R147).

Normal range: 0.8–1.4 mmol/L

Uses
Hypophosphataemia

Contraindications
Hypocalcaemia (further $\downarrow Ca^{2+}$)
Severe renal failure (risk of hyperphosphataemia)

Administration
10 ml potassium acid phosphate contains 10 mmol phosphate and 10 mmol potassium. Administer 1 ampoule (10 ml) (10 mmol phosphate) over 6 hours

Disodium hydrogen phosphate 21.49% w/v is an alternative to potassium phosphate (used in order to avoid potassium). 1 ampoule (10 ml) contains 6 mmol phosphate and 12 mmol sodium. Administer 2 ampoules (20 ml) (12 mmol phosphate) over 6 hours

The recommended dilution depends on whether it is given via the central (recommended) or peripheral route. For central venous route the dilution is to make up to 50 ml with sodium chloride 0.9% or glucose 5%. For the peripheral route, the dilution is to make up to 250 ml with sodium chloride 0.9% or glucose 5%

Alternatively phosphate polyfuser, 50 mmol/500 ml (also containing sodium 81 mmol and potassium 9.5 mmol). This is ready diluted for central or peripheral use. Moderate hypophosphataemia usually 7.5 ml/hour for 12 hours (equivalent to 9 mmol over 12 hours). For severe hypophosphataemia usual max. dose over 24 hours: 30 mmol up to 48 mmol may be given over 24 hours

- IV infusion

  Central IV route: 10–12 mmol phosphate made up to 50 ml with glucose 5% or sodium chloride 0.9%, given over 6 hours

  Peripheral IV route: 10–12 mmol phosphate made up to 250 ml with glucose 5% or sodium chloride 0.9%, given over 6 hours

PHOSPHATES

Do not give at >12 mmol over 6 hours
Repeat until plasma level is normal
Monitor serum calcium, phosphate, potassium and sodium daily

How not to use phosphates

Do not give at a rate >12 mmol over 6 hours
If using phosphate polyfuser, it is common to use only a small proportion of the bottle. Avoid overdosing the patient by ensuring the infusion is stopped when the prescribed volume has been infused.

Adverse effects

Hypocalcaemia, hypomagnesaemia, hyperkalaemia, hypernatraemia
Arrhythmias
Hypotension
Ectopic calcification

Cautions

Renal impairment
Concurrent use of potassium–sparing diuretics or ACE-I with potassium phosphate may result in hyperkalaemia
Concurrent use of corticosteroids with sodium phosphate may result in hypernatraemia

Organ failure

Renal: risk of hyperphosphataemia

Renal replacement therapy

Dialysed. Dose in all techniques is as per normal renal function. Treat hypophosphataemia only on the basis of measured serum levels

PIPERACILLIN + TAZOBACTAM (Tazocin)

Tazocin is a combination of piperacillin (a broad-spectrum penicillin) and tazobactam (a beta-lactamase inhibitor). It has activity against many Gram +ve, Gram −ve and anaerobic bacteria. Tazocin may act synergistically with aminoglycosides against Gram −ve organisms including *Pseudomonas aeruginosa*. However, it remains susceptible to chromosomal beta-lactamases expressed by Enterobacteriaceae such as *Enterobacter* spp. and *Citrobacter* spp. and is unreliable for organisms expressing extended spectrum beta-lactamases (ESBLs). Tazocin appears to have a lower propensity to cause superinfection with *Clostridium difficile* compared with fluoroquinolones and cephalosporins.

Uses
Intra-abdominal infection
Respiratory tract infection particularly nosocomial pneumonia
Severe upper urinary tract infection
Empirical therapy of a range of severe infections prior to availability of sensitivities
Febrile neutropenia (usually combined with an aminoglycoside)

Contraindications
Penicillin hypersensitivity
Cephalosporin hypersensitivity

Administration
Reconstitute 2.25 g with 10 ml WFI
Reconstitute 4.5 g with 20 ml WFI

- IV bolus: 2.25–4.5 g 6–8 hourly, given over 3–5 min
- IV infusion: dilute the reconstituted solution to at least 50 ml with 5% glucose or sodium chloride 0.9% given over 20–30 min

In renal impairment:

Infection	Dose (g)	Interval (h)
Mild–moderate	2.25	8
Moderate–serious	4.5	6–8

How not to use tazocin

CC (ml/min)	Dose (g)	Interval (h)
20–80	4.5	8
10–20	4.5	8–12
< 10	4.5	12

Not for intrathecal use (encephalopathy)
Do not mix in the same syringe with an aminoglycoside (efficacy of aminoglycoside reduced)

Adverse effects
Diarrhoea
Muscle pain or weakness
Hallucination
Convulsion (high dose or renal failure)

Cautions
Owing to the sodium content (~2 mmol/g), high doses may lead to hypernatraemia

Organ failure
Renal: reduce dose

Renal replacement therapy
No further dose modification is required during high-clearance CVVH; though in low-clearance techniques reduce dose to 4.5 g 12 hourly, dependent on clearance rate as described in Short Notes Renal Replacement Therapy (p. 300–303) and CC table given previously. HD dialysed, dose 4.5 g 12 hourly or 2.25 g 8 hourly. PD not dialysed, dose 4.5 g 12 hourly or 2.25 g 8 hourly

POTASSIUM CHLORIDE

Uses

Hypokalaemia

Contraindications
Severe renal failure
Severe tissue trauma
Untreated Addison's disease

Administration
IV infusion: 20 mmol in 50 ml sodium chloride 0.9% or glucose 5% via central line or undiluted via central line. Prefilled bags should preferably be used where possible

Potassium chloride 1.5 g (20 mmol K$^+$) in 10-ml ampoules

Concentrations greater than 40 mmol in 1 l should be administered centrally, though concentrations up to 80 mmol/l can be administered via a large peripheral vein

IV infusion: undiluted via central line
Do not give at >20 mmol/h

Monitor serum potassium regularly
Check serum magnesium in refractory hypokalaemia

How not to use potassium chloride
Do not infuse neat potassium chloride into a peripheral vein
Avoid extravasation and do not give IM or SC (severe pain and tissue necrosis)
Do not use neat potassium chloride to reconstitute antibiotics as this has inadvertently caused several deaths

Adverse effects
Muscle weakness
Arrhythmias
ECG changes

Cautions
Renal impairment
Concurrent use of potassium-sparing diuretics or ACE-I
Hypokalaemia is frequently associated with hypomagnesaemia

Organ failure
Renal: risk of hyperkalaemia

Renal replacement therapy
Potassium accumulates in renal failure. Removed by HD/HF/PD
Treat hypokalaemia only on the basis of measured serum levels

PROCHLORPERAZINE

A phenothiazine that inhibits the medullary chemoreceptor trigger zone.

Uses
Nausea and vomiting

Contraindications
Parkinson's disease

Administration
- IM/IV: 12.5 mg 6 hourly

  The IV route is not licensed

- PO/NG: acute attack − 20 mg then 10 mg after 2 hours; maintenance dose 5–10 mg 8–12 hourly

Adverse effects
Drowsiness
Postural hypotension, tachycardia
Extrapyramidal movements particularly in children, elderly and debilitated

Cautions
Concurrent use of other CNS depressants (enhanced sedation)

Organ failure
CNS: sedative effects increased
Hepatic: can precipitate coma
Renal: increase cerebral sensitivity

Renal replacement therapy
No further dose modification is required during renal replacement therapy

P

PROPOFOL

Propofol is an IV anaesthetic induction agent that is widely used as a sedative drug in the critically ill. Its major advantages are that it has a rapid onset of action and a rapid recovery even after prolonged infusion. Propofol 1% (10 mg/ml) and 2% (20 mg/ml) are formulated in intralipid. If the patient is receiving other IV lipid concurrently, a reduction in quantity should be made to account for the amount of lipid infused as propofol: 1 ml propofol 1% contains 0.1 g fat and 1 kcal.

Cremer, et al. (*The Lancet* 2001; **357**: 117–18) have suggested an association between long-term (>2 days) high-dose (>5 mg/kg/h) propofol infusion used for sedation and cardiac failure in adult patients with head injuries. All the seven patients who died developed metabolic acidosis, hyperkalaemia or rhabdomyolysis. Reports of similar suspected reactions, including hyperlipidaemia and hepatomegaly, were previously reported in children given propofol infusion for sedation in intensive care units, some with fatal outcome (MCA/CSM *Current Problems in Pharmacovigilance* 1992; 34).

Uses
Sedation, especially for weaning from other sedative agents (p. 266)
Status epilepticus (p. 270)

Contraindications
As an analgesic
Hypersensitivity to propofol, soybean oil or egg phosphatide (egg yolk)
Sedation of ventilated children aged 16 years or younger receiving intensive care

Administration
- IV bolus: 10–20 mg PRN
- IV infusion: up to 4 mg/kg/h

Titrate to desired level of sedation – assess daily
Measure serum triglycerides regularly
Contains no preservatives – discard after 12 h

How not to use propofol
Do not give in the same line as blood or blood products
Do not exceed recommended dose range for sedation (up to 4 mg/kg/h)

P

Adverse effects
Hypotension
Bradycardia
Apnoea
Pain on injection (minimised by mixing with lignocaine 1 mg for every 10 mg propofol)
Fat overload
Convulsions and myoclonic movements

Cautions
Epilepsy
Lipid disorders (risk of fat overload)
Egg allergy (most patients are allergic to the egg albumin – not egg yolk)

Organ failure
CNS: sedative effects increased
Cardiac: exaggerated hypotension

PROPOFOL

PROTAMINE

Available as a 1% (10 mg/ml) solution of protamine sulphate. Although it is used to neutralise the anticoagulant action of heparin and LMWH for the treatment of severe bleeding, if used in excess it has an anticoagulant effect. It should correct a prolonged APTR but it will only partially reverse LMWH.

Uses
Neutralise the anticoagulant action of heparin and LMWH

Contraindications
Hypersensitivity

Administration
1 ml 1% (10 mg) protamine is required to neutralise 1000 units of heparin given in the previous 15–30 min. Max. 50 mg protamine sulphate in any one dose; max. rate 5 mg/min. Slow IV injection 5 ml 1% over 10 min. APTT can be checked 15 minutes after a protamine sulphate dose. Once the APTT is corrected, recheck at 2 hours and then every 4–6 hours for the next 24 hours because of the possibility of heparin rebound

For heparin boluses
As more time elapses after the heparin injection, proportionally less protamine is required, i.e. if 30–60 mins have elapsed since the IV heparin bolus, then give 0.5–0.75 mg protamine sulphate per 100 units of heparin administered. If approximately 2 hours have elapsed, then give 0.25–0.375 mg per 100 units IV heparin

Ideally, the dosage should be guided by serial measurements of APTT/ACT and the rate guided by watching the direct arterial BP

For heparin infusions
As heparin has a short half-life it is usually sufficient to stop the IV infusion. Coagulation is mostly normal 4 hours after cessation. If severe bleeding, then only heparin given during the preceding few hours needs to be taken into account

The initial dose of protamine sulphate is 25–50 mg by slow IV (max. 5 mg/min). Consider using the lower dose if the infusion has been stopped for 1–2 hours and patient is still bleeding

Check APTT 15 minutes after a protamine sulphate dose. Once corrected, recheck at 2 hours and then every 4–6 hours for the next 24 hours because of the possibility of heparin rebound

How not to use protamine
Rapid IV bolus

Adverse effects
Hypersensitivity

Rapid IV administration – pulmonary vasoconstriction, $\downarrow$ left atrial pressure and hypotension

Cautions
Hypersensitivity (severe hypotension, may respond to fluid loading)

P

PROTAMINE

PYRIDOSTIGMINE (Mestinon)

Pyridostigmine is a cholinesterase inhibitor leading to prolongation of ACh action. This enhances neuromuscular transmission in voluntary and involuntary muscle in myasthenia gravis.

Uses
Myasthenia gravis

Administration
- Orally: 60–240 mg 4–6 hourly (maximum daily dose: 1.2 g)

When relatively large doses are taken it may be necessary to give atropine or other anticholinergic drugs to counteract the muscarinic effects

Contraindications
Bowel obstruction
Urinary obstruction

How not to use pyridostigmine
Excessive dosage may impair neuromuscular transmission and precipitates 'cholinergic crises' by causing a depolarising block. It is inadvisable to exceed a daily dose of 720 mg

Adverse effects
Increased sweating
Excess salivation
Nausea and vomiting
Abdominal cramp
Diarrhoea
Bradycardia
Hypotension
These muscarinic side-effects are antagonised by atropine

Cautions
Asthma

Organ failure
Renal: reduce dose

Renal replacement therapy
No further dose modification is required during renal replacement therapy

QUETIAPINE (Seroquel)

This is an atypical antipsychotic agent that antagonises a range of receptors, namely dopamine D_1, dopamine D_2, 5-HT_2, α_1-adrenoceptor and histamine-1. Although licensed for conditions such as acute schizophrenia, mania, depression and bipolar disorder, there is emerging experience of using this agent as an alternative to haloperidol in delirium, particularly in patients who have a prolonged QT interval. A case series (*Critical Care* 2011, **15**: R159) describes experience with a cohort of ICU patients. It has several attractive features: it is administered 12 hourly, has a relatively short half-life of 7 hours (12 hours for its active metabolite norquetiapine), is titratable and, importantly, has a lower incidence of QTc prolongation and fewer extrapyramidal symptoms than haloperidol.

Uses

Management of delirium in ICU patients (unlicensed), especially in prolonged QT interval as an alternative to benzodiazepines or in refractory or mixed delerium. Licensed indications: schizophrenia, mania, either alone or with mood stabilisers, depression in bipolar disorder, adjunctive treatment in major depressive disorder

Contraindications

Concomitant administration of cytochrome-P450 3A4 inhibitors such as HIV protease inhibitors, azole-antifungal agents, e.g. fluconazole, erythromycin, clarithromycin and nefazodone

Administration

- PO/NG initially 12.5 mg 12 hourly, titrated to response, typically to 25 mg 12 hourly for delirium and up to 200 mg 12 hourly. Max. licensed dose 375 mg 12 hourly
- Available as 25 mg, 100 mg, 150 mg, 200 mg and 300 mg tablets

Adverse effects

Most common: somnolence, dizziness, dry mouth, mild asthenia, constipation, tachycardia, orthostatic hypotension and dyspepsia
Elevated plasma triglyceride and cholesterol concentrations
QT prolongation
Hyperglycaemia
Withdrawal symptoms after long-term use
Seizures

Cautions

Hepatic enzyme inducers such as carbamazepine or phenytoin substantially decrease quetiapine plasma concentrations

Organ failure

Renal: no dose adjustment is required
Liver: titrate dose to response (lower dose may be necessary)

RAMIPRIL

ACE inhibitors have a beneficial role in all grades of heart failure, usually combined with a β-blocker and diuretics. Potassium-sparing diuretics should be discontinued before starting an ACE inhibitor because of the risk of hyperkalaemia. However, low-dose spironolactone may also be beneficial in severe heart failure, and when used together with an ACE inhibitor serum potassium needs to be monitored closely.

Uses
Hypertension
Heart failure

Contraindications
Aortic stenosis
HOCM
Porphyria
Angioedema (idiopathic or hereditary)
Known or suspected renal artery stenosis (co-existing diabetes, PVD, hypertension)

Administration
• Orally: 1.25 mg once daily, increased gradually to a maximum of 10 mg daily (daily doses of 2.5 mg or more may be taken in 1–2 divided doses)

Monitor:
BP
Serum potassium and creatinine

In renal impairment:

CC (ml/min)	Initial dose (mg)	Maximum once daily dose (mg)
0–30	1.25	5

Cautions
Risk of sudden and precipitous fall in BP in the following patients:

Dehydrated
Salt-depleted (Na^+ <130 mmol/l)
High-dose diuretics (>80 mg furosemide daily)

Concomitant NSAID (↑ risk of renal damage)
Concomitant potassium-sparing diuretics (hyperkalaemia)
Peripheral vascular disease or generalised atherosclerosis (risk of clinically silent renovascular disease)

Adverse effects
Hypotension
Tachycardia
Dry cough
Rash
Pancreatitis
Altered LFT
Acidosis
Angioedema

Organ failure
Renal: reduce dose; hyperkalaemia more common

Renal replacement therapy
No further dose modification is required during renal replacement therapy

RANITIDINE

It is a specific histamine H_2-antagonist that inhibits basal and stimulated secretion of gastric acid, reducing both the volume and the pH of the secretion.

Uses
Peptic ulcer disease
Prophylaxis of stress ulceration
Premedication in patients at risk of acid aspiration

Administration
- IV bolus: 50 mg 8 hourly

  Dilute to 20 ml with sodium chloride 0.9% or glucose 5% and give over 5 min

- Oral 150 mg 12 hourly

  For prevention of NSAID-induced GI toxicity, double the doses stated above

In renal impairment:

CC (ml/min)	Percentage of normal dose
<10	50–100

How not to use ranitidine
Do not give rapidly as IV bolus (bradycardia, arrhythmias)

Adverse effects
Hypersensitivity reactions
Bradycardia
Transient and reversible worsening of liver function tests
Reversible leukopenia and thrombocytopenia

Organ failure
Renal: reduce dose
Hepatic: reduce dose (increased risk of confusion)

Renal replacement therapy
No further dose modification is required during renal replacement therapy

REMIFENTANIL (Ultiva)

Remifentanil (*Ultiva*) is a potent, short-acting, selective μ opioid receptor agonist. In critical care, it has been used for sedation and analgesia in mechanically ventilated adult patients. The concept of analgesia-based sedation represents a move away from traditional analgesic/hypnotic-based sedation, and with appropriate training this may be an easier regimen to manage. Remifentanil is also licensed for use in general anaesthesia. It has an onset of action of approximately 1 min and quickly achieves steady state. It is metabolised rapidly by non-specific blood and tissue esterases into clinically inactive metabolites. Thus the terminal half-life of 10–20 min is independent of infusion duration and renal and hepatic dysfunction. Though more expensive than traditional analgesic/hypnotic-based regimens, some units use remifentanil particularly in patients with renal or hepatic dysfunction, to avoid accumulation and prolonged sedation. Other possible indications for remifentanil include overnight ventilation, tracheostomy and ready to wean, difficult weans (e.g. COPD, cardiovascular disease, obesity, problems of withdrawal following long-term sedation), head injuries or patients with low GCS requiring regular assessment, raised intracranial pressure (resistant to medical management) and to assess neurological function in mechanically ventilated patients.

Concerns around use of remifentanil include side-effects of hypotension and bradycardia, possible development of tolerance (common to all opioids) and the onset of pain on discontinuation of remifentanil.

Uses
Analgesia and sedation in mechanically ventilated adults. Trials have been conducted for up to 3 days of use.

Contraindications
Epidural and intrathecal use, as formulated with glycine
Hypersensitivity to fentanyl analogues

Administration
- IV: initially 0.1 μg/kg/min, evaluate after 5 min, if pain, anxiety or agitation or difficult to wake, then titrate infusion up or down with steps of 0.025 μg/kg/min (range 0.007–0.75 μg/kg/min). At a dose of 0.2 μg/kg/min, if the patient is in pain or ventilator intolerant, increase the infusion by additional steps of 0.025 μg/kg/min until adequate pain relief. At a dose of 0.2 μg/kg/min, if the patient is anxious or agitated then add a hypnotic agent, e.g. midazolam (bolus up to 0.03 mg/kg or initial infusion 0.03 mg/kg/h) or propofol (bolus up to 0.5 mg/kg or initial infusion 0.5 mg/kg/h)
- Additional analgesia will be required for ventilated patients undergoing stimulating procedures such as suctioning, wound dressing and physiotherapy. An infusion of 0.1 μg/kg/min should be maintained for at least 5 min prior to intervention. Further adjustments every 2–5 minutes in increments of 25–50% may be needed

- To extubate and discontinue remifentanil, titrate in stages to 0.1 µg/kg/min over 1 hour prior to extubation. After extubation, reduce infusion rate by 25% at least every 10 min till discontinuation. If residual pain is expected use alternative opioid

Reconstitute vial to 100 µg/ml, i.e. 5 mg vial with 50 ml, 2 mg with 20 ml, and 1 mg with 10 ml of diluent. Suitable diluents are WFI, glucose 5% or sodium chloride 0.9%

In obesity, use ideal body weight rather than actual weight

In the elderly, reduce initial dose by 50%

Due to the short half-life, a new syringe should be ready for use at the end of each infusion

How not to use remifentanil

Bolus doses are not recommended in the critical care setting. Not to be used as a sole induction agent

Adverse effects

- hypomagnesaemia
- bradycardia
- hypotension
- respiratory depression
- muscle rigidity
- dependency

Cautions

Upon discontinuation, the IV line should be cleared or removed to prevent subsequent inadvertent administration

Organ failure

Renal: no dose adjustment necessary

Hepatic: no dose adjustment, but in severe disease respiratory depression more common

Organ replacement therapy

Not removed by dialysis, so no dose adjustment required in renal replacement therapy

RIFAMPICIN

Rifampicin is active against a wide range of Gram +ve and Gram −ve organisms, but resistance readily emerges during therapy due to preexisting mutants present in most bacterial populations. It must therefore be used with a second antibiotic active against the target pathogen. Its major use is for therapy of tuberculosis.

Uses

In combination with vancomycin for:

* penicillin–resistant pneumococcal infections including meningitis
* serious Gram +ve infections including those caused by MRSA
* prosthetic device–associated infections

Legionnaires' disease (in combination with a macrolide antibiotic)
Prophylaxis of meningococcal meningitis and *Haemophilus influenzae* (type B) infection
Combination therapy for infections due to *Mycobacterium tuberculosis*

Contraindications

Porphyria
Jaundice

Administration

* Serious Gram +ve infections (in combination with vancomycin)
* Legionnaires' disease (in combination with a macrolide antibiotic)

    Oral or IV: 600 mg 12 hourly

* Prophylaxis of meningococcal meningitis infection

    Oral or IV: 600 mg 12 hourly for 2 days
    Child 10 mg/kg (under 1 year, 5 mg/kg) 12 hourly for 2 days

* Prophylaxis of *Haemophilus influenzae* (type b) infection

    Oral or IV: 600 mg once daily for 4 days
    Child 1–3 months 10 mg/kg once daily for 4 days, over 3 months 20 mg/kg once daily for 4 days (maximum 600 mg daily)

IV formulation is available as *Rifadin*
Reconstitute with the solvent provided, then dilute with 500 ml of glucose 5%, sodium chloride 0.9% or Hartmann's solution given over 2–3 hours

Monitor: FBC, U&E, LFT

R

Adverse effects
GI symptoms (nausea, vomiting, diarrhoea)
Bodily secretions (urine, saliva) coloured orange-red
Abnormal LFT
Haemolytic anaemia
Thrombocytopenic purpura
Renal failure

Cautions
Discolours soft contact lenses
Women on oral contraceptive pills will need other means of contraception

Organ failure
Hepatic: avoid or do not exceed 8 mg/kg daily (impaired elimination)

SALBUTAMOL

S

Uses
Reverses bronchospasm

Administration
- Nebuliser: 2.5–5 mg 6 hourly, undiluted (if prolonged delivery time desirable then dilute with sodium chloride 0.9% only)
  For patients with chronic bronchitis and hypercapnia, oxygen in high concentration can be dangerous, and nebulisers should be driven by air
- IV: 5 mg made up to 50 ml with glucose 5% (100 μg/ml)
  Rate: 200–1200 μg/h (2–12 ml/h)

How not to use salbutamol
For nebuliser: do not dilute in anything other than sodium chloride 0.9% (hypotonic solution may cause bronchospasm)

Adverse effects
Tremor
Tachycardia
Paradoxical bronchospasm (stop giving if suspected)
Potentially serious hypokalaemia (potentiated by concomitant treatment with aminophylline, steroids, diuretics and hypoxia)

Cautions
Thyrotoxicosis
In patients already receiving large doses of other sympathomimetic drugs

SALBUTAMOL

SILDENAFIL

Sildenafil (Viagra, Revatio), epoprostenol (Flolan), bosentan (Tracleer) and sitaxentan (Thelin) are licensed for the treatment of pulmonary hypertension. Epoprostenol and sildenafil are both available for intravenous use. Sildenafil is a potent and selective inhibitor of cyclic guanosine monophosphate (cGMP) specific phosphodiesterase type 5 (PDE5), the enzyme that is responsible for degradation of cGMP. Apart from the presence of this enzyme in the corpus cavernosum of the penis, PDE5 is also present in the pulmonary vasculature. Sildenafil, therefore, increases cGMP within pulmonary vascular smooth muscle cells, resulting in relaxation. In patients with pulmonary arterial hypertension this can lead to vasodilatation of the pulmonary vascular bed and, to a lesser degree, vasodilatation in the systemic circulation.

Uses
Pulmonary hypertension

Contraindications
Recent stroke or MI
Severe hypotension (SBP <90 mmHg)
Severe hepatic impairment (Child–Pugh class C)
Avoid concomitant use of nitrates, ketoconazole, itraconazole and ritonavir

Administration
- Orally: 20 mg 8 hourly

    Renal impairment: 20 mg 12 hourly
    Hepatic impairment (Child–Pugh class A and B): 20 mg 12 hourly

- IV bolus: 10 mg 8 hourly. Ready diluted. Vial contains 10 mg (as citrate) in 12.5 ml (0.8 mg/ml). 10 mg IV has equivalent effect to 20 mg orally.

Adverse effects
GI disturbances
Dry mouth
Flushing
Headaches
Back and limb pain
Visual disturbances
Hearing loss
Pyrexia

Cautions
Hypotension (avoid if SBP <90 mmHg)
Dehydration
Left ventricular outflow obstruction
IHD
Predisposition to priapism
Bleeding disorders
Active peptic ulceration
Hepatic impairment (avoid if severe)
Renal impairment (reduce dose)

SODIUM VALPROATE (Epilim)

Sodium valproate is used to treat epilepsy. The IV route is chosen only when the oral/nasogastric route is unavailable. The therapeutic range for trough plasma valproic acid levels is 40–100 mg/l (278–694 μmol/l), though there is a less reliable correlation between the level and efficacy. The oral form is available as a liquid (200 mg/5 ml), which is useful for nasogastric administration, and tablets, crushable tablets and in modified release formulations. Sodium valproate should not be confused with valproic acid (as semi-sodium valproate), which is licensed for acute mania. Valproate overdose can cause hyperammonaemia encephalopathy, which can be treated with carnitine (IV 500 mg/m^2 twice daily) (see *Critical Care* 2005; **9**: 431–40)

Uses
All forms of epilepsy, including emergency management

Administration
For conversion of oral to IV doses, the same daily dose is used in divided doses administered over 3–5 min

Initiating IV valproate: 400–800 mg (up to 10 mg/kg), then IV infusion of up to 2.5 g maximum

To prepare, reconstitute 400 mg vial with 4 ml diluent provided and further dilute to a convenient volume with sodium chloride 0.9% or glucose 5%. It may be administered as a bolus over 3–5 min or as a continuous infusion

Oral: usually 20–30 mg/kg/day in two divided doses

Adverse effects
Transient raised LFTs
Severe liver dysfunction, which can be fatal
Hyperammonaemia and hyponatraemia
Rarely exanthematous rash

Cautions
Pancreatitis
Liver toxicity

Sodium valproate is eliminated mainly through the kidneys, partly in the form of ketone bodies; this may give false positives in urine testing. Sodium valproate concentrations are reduced by carbamazepine and phenytoin. Valproate increases or sometimes decreases phenytoin levels, and increases levels of lamotrigine

Organ failure
Renal: no dose adjustment required
Hepatic: avoid if possible; hepatotoxicity and hepatic failure may occasionally occur

SPIRONOLACTONE

S

Spironolactone is a potassium-sparing diuretic, which acts by antagonising aldosterone. Low doses of spironolactone have been shown to benefit patients with severe congestive heart failure who are already receiving an ACE inhibitor and a diuretic. It is also of value in the treatment of oedema and ascites in cirrhosis of the liver.

Uses
Congestive heart failure
Oedema and ascites in liver cirrhosis

Contraindications
Hyperkalaemia
Hyponatraemia
Severe renal failure
Addison's disease

Administration
- Congestive heart failure

    Orally: 25–50 mg once daily

- Oedema and ascites in liver cirrhosis

    Orally: 100–400 mg once daily

If IV route is needed, use potassium canrenoate (unlicensed drug). Conversion: potassium canrenoate 140 mg is equivalent to spironolactone 100 mg. Administer by IV bolus via a large vein at a maximum rate of 100 mg/min, otherwise administer via IV infusion in 250 ml of glucose 5% over 90 min

Monitor: serum sodium, potassium and creatinine

Adverse effects
Confusion
Hyperkalaemia (unlikely to occur with congestive heart failure dose)
Hyponatraemia
Abnormal LFT
Gynaecomastia (usually reversible)
Rashes

Cautions
Porphyria
Renal impairment (risk of hyperkalaemia)
Concurrent use of:

- ACE inhibitor (risk of hyperkalaemia)
- angiotensin-II antagonist (risk of hyperkalaemia)
- digoxin ($\uparrow$ plasma concentration of digoxin)
- ciclosporin (risk of hyperkalaemia)
- lithium ($\uparrow$ plasma concentration of lithium)

Organ failure
Renal: risk of hyperkalaemia; use with caution in severe renal failure
Hepatic: may precipitate encephalopathy

Renal replacement therapy
CVVH not dialysable, dose as in CC 10–20 ml/min, i.e. half normal dose. HD/PD not dialysable, use with caution; 25 mg three times per week appears safe

SUCRALFATE

A complex of aluminium hydroxide and sulphated sucrose. It acts by protecting the mucosa from acid–pepsin attack.

Uses
Prophylaxis of stress ulceration

Contraindications
Severe renal impairment (CC <10 ml/min)

Administration
• Orally: 1 g suspension 4 hourly

   Stop sucralfate when enteral feed commences

How not to use sucralfate
Do not give with enteral feed (risk of bezoar formation)
Do not give ranitidine concurrently (may need acid environment to work)

Adverse effects
Constipation
Diarrhoea
Hypophosphataemia

Cautions
Renal impairment (neurological adverse effects due to aluminium toxicity)
Risk of bezoar formation and potential intestinal obstruction
Interferes with absorption of quinolone antibiotics, phenytoin and digoxin when given orally

Organ failure
Renal: aluminium may accumulate

Renal replacement therapy
CVVH not dialysable, dependent on clearance rate as described in Short Notes Renal Replacement Therapy (p. 300–303), for CC 10–20 ml/min, i.e. half normal dose 2–4 g daily. HD/PD not dialysable CC <10 ml/min, i.e. 2–4 g daily

SUGAMMADEX (Bridion)

This drug is used for rapid reversal of neuromuscular blockade induced by rocuronium or vecuronium. It forms a tight one-to-one complex with rocuronium/vecuronium, encapsulating the drug in the plasma and hence reducing its concentration at the neuromuscular junction and rapidly terminating block. Unlike acetylcholinesterase inhibitors, e.g. neostigmine, sugammadex can be given for immediate reversal without the need for partial recovery. Having no effect on acetylcholinesterase, concomitant anticholinergic drugs, e.g. glycopyrrolate, are not required with sugammadex. Use of this drug replaces the use of suxamethonium, which can cause anaphylactic/allergic reactions, myalgia, cardiac arrest and induce malignant hyperthermia. However, it is substantially more expensive than alternative agents, which may be prohibitive for routine reversal.

Uses

Emergency reversal of neuromuscular blockade where standard reversal is likely to be too slow, i.e. 'cannnot intubate, cannot ventilate' scenarios

Administration

The dose is dependent on the level of neuromuscular blockade to be reversed rather than the anaesthetic regimen

For routine reversal: if recovery has reached at least 1–2 post-tetanic counts (PTC), the dose is 4 mg/kg

If spontaneous recovery has reached at least the appearance of T2, the dose is 2 mg/kg

If re-occurrence of blockade occurs postoperatively, a repeat dose of 4 mg/kg may be given with close monitoring for return of neuromuscular function

Administer as an IV bolus over 10 seconds. It can be injected into an IV line of infusions of sodium chloride 0.9%, glucose 5% or Hartmann's solution. Flush with sodium chloride 0.9% after use

At least a 24-hour interval must be observed before re-administration of vecuronium or rocuronium after sugammadex administration. If further neuromuscular blockade is required, a non-steroid neuromuscular blocking agent must be used

Adverse effects

Hypersensitivity reactions
Bronchospasm

Displacement interactions

These can occur as vecuronium or rocuronium may be displaced from sugammadex, carrying a risk of re-occurrence of blockade. This may occur with:

Toremifine: patients who have received this drug on the day of operation may have delayed recovery of the T4/T1 ratio to 0.9

Fusidic acid injection: patients receiving this in the pre-operative period may have delayed recovery of the T4/T1 ratio to 0.9 Cautions

In those with an increased bleeding risk, the anaesthetist needs to make a risk/benefit assessment before use in relation to history of bleeding episodes and type of surgery. High bleeding risk includes: warfarin with INR>3.4, anticoagulant use with those receiving a dose of sugammadex 16 mg/kg, pre-existing coagulopathies, hereditary vitamin K-dependent clotting factor deficiencies

Sugammadex can reduce the effect of hormonal contraceptives – extra precautions are necessary – one 4 mg/kg dose is similar to missing one oral contraceptive dose

Organ failure

Renal: mild-moderate impairment – no change

CrCl <30 ml/min not recommended

Hepatic: no adjustment required, in severe impairment, use with caution as no studies in this group

Renal replacement therapy

Unchanged but haemofiltration rate should be at least 2 l/h

How not to use sugammadex

Do not reuse rocuronium/vecuronium within 24 hours of sugammadex use

SUXAMETHONIUM

The only depolarising neuromuscular blocker available in the UK. It has a rapid onset of action (45–60 s) and a short duration of action (5 min). Breakdown is dependent on plasma pseudocholinesterase. It is best to keep the ampoule in the fridge to prevent a gradual loss of activity due to spontaneous hydrolysis.

Uses
Agent of choice for:

- rapid tracheal intubation as part of a rapid sequence induction
- for procedures requiring short periods of tracheal intubation, e.g. cardioversion
- management of severe post-extubation laryngospasm unresponsive to gentle positive pressure ventilation

Contraindications
History of malignant hyperpyrexia (potent trigger)
Hyperkalaemia (expect a further increase in K$^+$ level by 0.5–1.0 mmol/l)
Patients where exaggerated increase in K$^+$ (>1.0 mmol/l) are expected:

- severe burns
- extensive muscle damage
- disuse atrophy
- paraplegia and quadriplegia
- peripheral neuropathy, e.g. Guillain–Barré

Administration
As a rapid sequence induction: 1.0–1.5 mg/kg IV bolus, after 3 min pre-oxygenation with 100% O_2 and a sleep dose of induction agent

Apply cricoid pressure until tracheal intubation confirmed. Intubation possible within 1 min. Effect normally lasting <5 min

Repeat dose of 0.25–0.5 mg/kg may be given. Atropine or glycopyrollate should be given at the same time to avoid bradycardia/asystole

How not to use suxamethonium
In the conscious patient
By persons not trained to intubate the trachea

Adverse effects
Malignant hyperpyrexia
Hyperkalaemia
Transient increase in IOP and ICP
Muscle pain
Myotonia
Bradycardia, especially after repeated dose

S

Cautions
Digoxin (may cause arrhythmias)
Myasthenia gravis (resistant to usual dose)
Penetrating eye injury (IOP may cause loss of globe contents)
Prolonged block in:

- patients taking aminoglycoside antibiotics, magnesium
- myasthenic syndrome
- pseudocholinesterase deficiency (inherited or acquired)

Organ failure
Hepatic: prolonged apnoea (reduced synthesis of pseudocholinesterase)

TEICOPLANIN

This glycopeptide antibiotic, like vancomycin, has bactericidal activity against both aerobic and anaerobic Gram +ve bacteria: *Staphylococcus aureus*, including MRSA, *Streptococcus* spp., *Listeria* spp. and *Clostridium* spp. It is only bacteriostatic for most *Enterococcus* spp. It does not cause red man syndrome through histamine release and is less nephrotoxic than vancomycin. However, due to the variation between patients, effective therapeutic levels for severe infections may not be reached for a number of days using the most commonly recommended dosage schedules. Serum monitoring of pre-dose levels is recommended, particularly for severe infections.

In the UK resistance is well recognised in enterococci and coagulase-negative staphylococci and, more worryingly, is now emerging in *S. aureus*.

Uses
Serious Gram +ve infections:

- prophylaxis and treatment of infective endocarditis (usually combined with gentamicin)
- dialysis-associated peritonitis
- infection caused by MRSA
- prosthetic device infections due to coagulase-negative staphylococci
- alternative to penicillins and cephalosporins where patients are allergic

Contraindications
Hypersensitivity

Administration
IV bolus: 400 mg 12 hourly for 3 doses, then 400 mg daily. Give over 3–5 min

In obesity, use 6 mg/kg per dose (rounded to the nearest 100 mg) rather than 400 mg

Reconstitute with WFI supplied. Gently roll the vial between the hands until powder is completely dissolved. Shaking the solution will cause the formation of foam. If the solution becomes foamy allow to stand for 15 min

Monitor: FBC, U&E, LFT
　　　　　Serum pre-dose teicoplanin level

Pre-dose (trough) serum concentration should not be <10 mg/l
For severe infections, trough serum concentration >20 mg/l is recommended. Levels are not essential for treatment

In renal impairment: dose reduction not necessary until day 4, then reduce dose as below:

CC (ml/min)	Dose (mg)	Interval
20–25	400	every day
10–20	400	every 24–48 h
<10	400	every 48–72 h

How not to use teicoplanin
Do not mix teicoplanin and aminoglycosides in the same syringe

Adverse effects
Raised LFTs
Hypersensitivity
Blood disorders
Ototoxic
Nephrotoxic

Cautions
Vancomycin sensitivity
Renal/hepatic impairment
Concurrent use of ototoxic and nephrotoxic drugs

Organ failure
Renal: reduce dose

Renal replacement therapy
CVVH unknown dialysability, dose dependent on clearance rate as described in Short Notes Renal Replacement Therapy, (p. 300–303), and CC table given previously. HD/PD not dialysable, dose 400 mg 12 hourly for 3 doses then 400 mg every 48–72 hours. Can measure levels for therapy optimisation but is not essential

TERLIPRESSIN

Oesophageal varices are enlarged blood vessels that form in the stomach or oesophagus as a complication of liver disease. When administered in bleeding oesophageal varices, terlipressin (Glypressin and Variquel) is broken down to release lysine vasopressin, which causes vasoconstriction of these vessels thereby reducing the bleeding. In addition, terlipressin may have a role in the treatment of hepatorenal syndrome, by increasing renal perfusion. Terlipressin can also be used in resistant septic shock, in addition to noradrenaline.

Uses
Bleeding oesophageal varices
Resistant high-output septic shock
Hepatorenal syndrome

Contraindications
Pregnancy

Administration
- Varices

    IV bolus: 2 mg, then 1–2 mg every 4–6 hourly, for up to 3 days

- Resistant high-output septic shock (unlicensed indication)

    IV 0.25 mg bolus, repeated up to 4 times with 20-min intervals between doses or IV infusion (unlicensed) 0.1 mg/h (can increase to 0.3 mg/h). Will take 20 min for first effect. The infusion can be made up with 1 mg in 5 ml with the diluent provided or the ready diluted solution

- Hepatorenal syndrome (unlicensed indication)

    IV bolus: 0.5–1 mg 6 hourly

Terlipressin is available in two brands and three presentations: Glypressin 1 mg/8.5 ml solution (stored in fridge), Glypressin and Variquel both 1 mg with 5 ml diluent (stored at room temperature)

Monitor: BP
            Serum sodium and potassium
            Fluid balance

Adverse effects
Abdominal cramps
Headache
Raised blood pressure

Cautions
Hypertension
Arrhythmias
Ischaemic heart disease

Organ failure
Renal: no dose reduction needed

THIOPENTONE

Thiopentone is a barbiturate that is used widely as an IV anaesthetic agent. It also has cerebroprotective and anticonvulsant activities. Awakening from a bolus dose is rapid due to redistribution, but hepatic metabolism is slow and sedative effects may persist for 24 hours. Repeated doses or infusion has a cumulative effect. Available in 500 mg ampoules or 2.5 g vial, which is dissolved in 20 or 100 ml WFI respectively to make a 2.5% solution.

Uses
Induction of anaesthesia
Status epilepticus (p. 270)

Contraindications
Airway obstruction
Previous hypersensitivity
Status asthmaticus
Porphyria

Administration
- IV bolus: 2.5–4 mg/kg. After injecting a test dose of 2 ml, if no pain, give the rest over 20–30 s until loss of eyelash reflex. Give further 50–100 mg if necessary

  Reduce dose and inject more slowly in the elderly, patients with severe hepatic and renal impairment, and in hypovolaemic and shocked patients. In obese patients, dosage should be based on lean body mass

How not to use thiopentone
Do not inject into an artery (pain and ischaemic damage)
Do not inject solution >2.5% (thrombophlebitis)

Adverse effects
Hypersensitivity reactions (1:14 000–35 000)
Coughing, laryngospasm
Bronchospasm (histamine release)
Respiratory depression and apnoea
Hypotension, myocardial depression
Tachycardia, arrhythmias
Tissue necrosis from extravasation

Cautions
Hypovolaemia
Septic shock
Elderly (reduce dose)
Asthma

Organ failure
CNS: sedative effects increased
Cardiac: exaggerated hypotension and ↓ cardiac output
Respiratory: ↑ respiratory depression
Hepatic: enhanced and prolonged sedative effect. Can precipitate coma
Renal: increased cerebral sensitivity

T

THIOPENTONE

TICARCILLIN + CLAVULANIC ACID (Timentin)

Timentin is a broad-spectrum antibiotic with bactericidal activity against a wide range of Gram +ve and Gram −ve aerobic and anaerobic bacteria. It contains ticarcillin and clavulanic acid. The presence of clavulanic acid extends the spectrum of activity of ticarcillin to include many β-lactamase-producing bacteria normally resistant to ticarcillin and other β-lactam antibiotics. Timentin acts synergistically with aminoglycosides against a number of organisms, including *Pseudomonas*.

Timentin is not active against MRSA.

Uses
Intra-abdominal infections including peritonitis
Pneumonia
Urinary tract infections
Skin and soft tissue infections

Contraindications
Hypersensitivity to β-lactam antibiotics (penicillins and cephalosporins)

Administration
• IV infusion: 3.2 g 6–8 hourly (maximum 3.2 g 4 hourly)

Reconstitute 3.2-g vial with 100 ml WFI or glucose 5%, given over 30 min

In renal impairment:

CC (ml/min)	Dose (g)	Interval (h)
>30	3.2	8
10–30	1.6	8
<10	1.6	12

How not use Timentin
Do not give IV infusion over longer than 40 min, as this may result in subtherapeutic concentrations

Adverse effects
Hypersensitivity
Hypokalaemia
False-positive Coombs' test
Thrombocytopenia
Prolonged prothrombin time

Cautions
Renal impairment (reduce dose)
Each 3.2 g vial of Timentin contains 15.9 mmol of sodium. A typical
daily dose regime may contain over 60 mmol Na^+

Renal replacement therapy
CVVH unknown dialysability, dependent on clearance rate as described
in Short Notes Renal Replacement Therapy (p. 300–303) and CC
table given previously. HD dialysed, dose 1.6 g every 12 hours. PD not
dialysed, dose 1.6 g 12 hourly

T

TICARCILLIN + CLAVULANIC ACID (Timentin)

TIGECYCLINE (Tygacil)

Tigecycline is a glycylcycline antibiotic (structurally similar to tetracyclines) with a broad-spectrum bactericidal activity against a wide range of Gram +ve and Gram −ve aerobic and anaerobic bacteria. It acts by inhibiting protein translocation in bacteria. Tigecycline is not active against *Pseudomonas aeruginosa*. The primary route of elimination is biliary excretion of unchanged tigecycline.

Uses
Intra-abdominal infections including peritonitis
Skin and soft tissue infections

Contraindications
Hypersensitivity to tetracycline
Pregnancy and lactating women (permanent tooth discoloration in foetuses)
Children and adolescents under the age of 18 years (permanent tooth discoloration)

Administration
- IV infusion: initial dose of 100 mg, followed by 50 mg 12 hourly, given over 30–60 min, for 5–14 days

Reconstitute the 50 mg vial with either 5 ml sodium chloride 0.9% or 5 ml glucose 5%. For a 100 mg dose, reconstitute using two vials. Then add the reconstituted solution to 100 ml sodium chloride 0.9% or 100 ml glucose 5% and give over 30–60 min

In severe hepatic impairment (Child–Pugh C): initial dose of 100 mg, followed by 25 mg 12 hourly

Adverse effects
Hypersensitivity
Acute pancreatitis
Elevated LFTs
Hyperphosphataemia
Prolonged APPT and PT
Clostridium difficile-associated diarrhoea

Cautions
Severe hepatic impairment (reduce dose)
Concurrent use of warfarin (increased INR)

Renal replacement therapy
No dosage adjustment required

TRANEXAMIC ACID

Tranexamic acid is an antifibrinolytic employed in blood conservation. It acts by inhibiting plasminogen activation.

Uses
Uncontrolled haemorrhage following prostatectomy or dental extraction in haemophiliacs
Haemorrhage due to thrombolytic therapy
Haemorrhage associated with DIC with predominant activation of the fibrinolytic system

Contraindications
Thrombo-embolic disease
DIC with predominant activation of coagulation system

Administration
- Uncontrolled haemorrhage following prostatectomy or dental extraction in haemophiliacs

  Slow IV: 500–1000 mg 8 hourly, given over 5–10 min (100 mg/min)

- Haemorrhage due to thrombolytic therapy

  Slow IV: 10 mg/kg, given at 100 mg/min

- Haemorrhage associated with DIC with predominant activation of the fibrinolytic system (prolonged PT, ↓ fibrinogen, ↑ fibrinogen degradation products)

  Slow IV: 1000 mg over 10 min, single dose usually sufficient. Heparin should be instigated to prevent fibrin deposition

In renal impairment:

CC (ml/min)	Dose (mg/kg)	Interval
20–50	10	12 hourly
10–20	10	every 12–24 h
<10	5	every 12–24 h

How not to use tranexamic acid
Rapid IV bolus

Adverse effects
Dizziness on rapid IV injection
Hypotension on rapid IV injection

Cautions
Renal impairment (reduce dose)

Organ failure
Renal: reduce dose

T

Renal replacement therapy
CVVH unknown dialysability, dose dependent on clearance rate as described in Short Notes Renal Replacement Therapy (pp. 300–303) as in CC table given previously. HD/PD unknown dialysability, CC <10 ml/min, i.e. 5 mg/kg every 12–24 hours

TRANEXAMIC ACID

VANCOMYCIN (Vancocin)

This glycopeptide antibiotic has bactericidal activity against aerobic and anaerobic Gram +ve bacteria, including MRSA. It is only bacteriostatic for most enterococci. It is used for therapy of *Clostridium difficile*-associated diarrhoea unresponsive to metronidazole, for which it has to be given by mouth. It is not significantly absorbed from the gut.

Serum level monitoring is required to ensure therapeutic levels are achieved and to limit toxicity. Successful treatment of MRSA infections requires levels above the traditionally recommended range. Under-dosing and problems associated with the sampling and the timing of serum level monitoring are problems that may result in decreased efficacy of vancomycin in the treatment of infection. The efficacy of vancomycin depends on the time for which the serum level exceeds the MIC (minimum inhibitory concentration) for the micro-organism rather than the attainment of high peak levels. Administration of vancomycin as a continuous IV infusion is therefore an ideal method of administration for optimum efficacy. Once the infusion reaches a steady state, the timing for serum level monitoring is not crucial, and samples can be taken at any time.

Vancomycin-resistant strains of enterococcus (VRE) are well recognised in the UK. Resistance also occurs less commonly in coagulase-negative staphylococci and is starting to emerge in rare isolates of *Staphylococcus aureus*.

Uses

C. difficile-associated diarrhoea via the oral route

Serious Gram +ve infections:

- prophylaxis and treatment of infective endocarditis (usually combined with gentamicin)
- dialysis-associated peritonitis
- infection caused by MRSA
- prosthetic device infections due to coagulase-negative staphylococci
- alternative to penicillins and cephalosporins where patients are allergic

Contraindications

Hypersensitivity

Administration

- *C. difficile*-associated diarrhoea

Orally: 125 mg 6 hourly for 7–10 days

For NG administration, the 500 mg reconstituted vial can be used nasogastrically for the four daily doses, otherwise 125 mg capsules can be used

Levels
Pre-dose (trough) level

- 10–15 mg/l
- 15–20 mg/l used for less sensitive strains of MRSA and severe or deep-seated infections, i.e. MRSA pneumonia, osteomyelitis, endocarditis, bacteraemia

Post-dose (peak) level
Post (peak) levels are not required to be measured

Adjustment of according to levels	
Pre-dose (trough) level	Maintenance dose adjustment
<5 mg/l	Move up to 2 levels from current dosing schedule
5–10 mg/l	Move up 1 level from current dosing schedule
10–15 mg/l	Continue at current dose
>15–20 mg/l	Continue at current dose
>20–25 mg/l	Move down 1 level without omitting any doses
>25 mg/l	Omit next dose & decrease by 2 levels from current dosing schedule
>30 mg/l	Seek advice

For continuous IV infusion (see Appendix J)

Monitor: renal function

Serum vancomycin levels (p. 250)

How not to use vancomycin
Rapid IV infusion (severe hypotension, thrombophlebitis)
Not for IM administration

Adverse effects
Following IV use:

- severe hypotension
- flushing of upper body ('red man' syndrome)
- ototoxic and nephrotoxic
- blood disorders
- hypersensitivity
- rashes

V

Cautions

Concurrent use of:

- aminoglycosides – ↑ ototoxicity and nephrotoxicity
- loop diuretics – ↑ ototoxicity

Organ failure

Renal: reduce dose

Renal replacement therapy

CVVH dialysed, dependent on clearance rate as described in Short Notes Renal Replacement Therapy (p. 300–303) and maintenance dose table given previously. For continuous vancomycin infusions, consult local guidance for dosing in CVVH. HD/PD not dialysable, dose as in CC <10 ml/min, i.e. 500 mg–1 g IV every 48–96 hours. For oral/enteral treatment, no dose adjustment is needed in renal replacement therapy as insignificant absorption occurs

VASOPRESSIN

Vasopressin (antidiuretic hormone, ADH) controls water excretion in kidneys via V2 receptors and produces constriction of vascular smooth muscle via V1 receptors. In normal subjects vasopressin infusion has no effect on blood pressure but has been shown to significantly increase blood pressure in septic shock. The implication is that in septic shock there is a deficiency in endogenous vasopressin, and this has been confirmed by direct measurement of endogenous vasopressin in patients with septic shock requiring vasopressors. *In vitro* studies show that catecholamines and vasopressin work synergistically.

Anecdotally, use of 3 units per hour is usually very effective and not associated with a reduction in urine output.

As its pseudonym antidiuretic hormone implies, vasopressin infusion might be expected to decrease urine output, but the opposite is the case at doses required in septic shock. This may be due to an increase in blood pressure and therefore perfusion pressure. It is also worth noting that, whereas noradrenaline constricts the afferent renal arteriole, vasopressin does not, so may be beneficial in preserving renal function. It has been shown that doses as high as 0.1 units/min (6 units/h) do reduce renal blood flow, so should be avoided. A dose of 0.04 units/min (2.4 units/h) is often efficacious in septic shock and does not reduce renal blood flow. The VAAST study (*N Engl J Med* 2008; **358**: 877–87) found that low-dose vasopressin (0.01–0.03 units/min) in addition to noradrenaline did not reduce mortality compared with noradrenaline alone. However, benefit was seen in less severe septic shock, where mortality was lower in the vasopressin group. The less severe group were identified as those stabilised on noradrenaline at doses of 5–15 μg/min.

Vasopressin does not cause vasoconstriction in the pulmonary or cerebral vessels, presumably due to an absence of vasopressin receptors. It does cause vasoconstriction in the splanchnic circulation, hence the use of vasopressin in bleeding oesophageal varices. The dose required in septic shock is much lower than that required for variceal bleeding.

Uses
In septic shock: reserve its use in cases where the noradrenaline dose exceeds 0.3 μg/kg/min (unlicensed)

Contraindications
Vascular disease, especially coronary artery disease

Administration
IV infusion: 1–4 units/h

Dilute 20 units (1 ml ampoule of argipressin) in 20 ml glucose 5% (1 unit/ml) and start at 1 unit/h, increasing to a maximum of 4 units/h

Do not stop the noradrenaline, as it works synergistically with vasopressin. As the patient's condition improves, the vasopressin should be weaned down and off before the noradrenaline is stopped

Available as argipressin (Pitressin)
Stored in fridge between 2 and 8°C

How not to use vasopressin
Doses in excess of 5 units/h

Adverse effects
Abdominal cramps
Myocardial ischaemia
Peripheral ischaemia

Cautions
Heart failure
Hypertension

V

VASOPRESSIN

VECURONIUM

A non-depolarising neuromuscular blocker with minimal cardiovascular effects. It is metabolised in the liver to inactive products and has a duration of action of 20–30 min. Dose may have to be reduced in hepatic/renal failure.

Uses
Muscle paralysis

Contraindications
Airway obstruction
To facilitate tracheal intubation in patients at risk of regurgitation

Administration
- Initial dose: 100 µg/kg IV
- Incremental dose: 20–30 µg/kg according to response

Monitor with peripheral nerve stimulator

How not to use vecuronium
As part of a rapid sequence induction
In the conscious patient
By persons not trained to intubate the trachea

Cautions
Breathing circuit (disconnection)
Prolonged use (disuse muscle atrophy)

Organ failure
Hepatic: prolonged duration of action
Renal: prolonged duration of action

VERAPAMIL

A calcium–channel blocker that prolongs the refractory period of the AV node.

Uses
SVT
AF
Atrial flutter

Contraindications
Sinus bradycardia
Heart block
Congestive cardiac failure
VT/VF – may produce severe hypotension or cardiac arrest
WPW syndrome

Administration
- IV bolus: 5–10 mg over 2 min, may repeat with 5 mg after 10 min if required

IV infusion (unlicensed): SVT bolus dose (as previously) then continuous infusion of 5 mg/hr
Continuous ECG and BP monitoring
Decrease dose in liver disease and in the elderly

How not to use verapamil
Do not use in combination with β-blockers (bradycardia, heart failure, heart block, asystole)

Adverse effects
Bradycardia
Hypotension
Heart block
Asystole

Cautions
Sick sinus syndrome
Hypertrophic obstructive cardiomyopathy
Increased risk of toxicity from theophylline and digoxin

Organ failure
Hepatic: reduce dose

VITAMIN K (PHYTOMENADIONE)

Vitamin K is necessary for the production of prothrombin, factors VII, IX and X. It is found primarily in leafy green vegetables and is additionally synthesised by bacteria that colonise the gut. Because it is fat-soluble, it requires bile salts for absorption from the gut. Patients with biliary obstruction or hepatic disease may become deficient. Vitamin K deficiency is not uncommon in hospitalised patients because of poor diet, parenteral nutrition, recent surgery, antibiotic therapy or uraemia.

Uses
Liver disease
Reversal of warfarin

Contraindications
Hypersensitivity
Reversal of warfarin when need for re-warfarinisation likely (use FFP)

Administration
- Konakion® (0.5-ml ampoule containing 1 mg phytomenadione)

  IV bolus: 1–10 mg, give over 3–5 min
  Contains polyethoxylated castor oil which has been associated with anaphylaxis; should not be diluted

- Konakion® MM (1-ml ampoule containing 10 mg phytomenadione in a colloidal formulation)

  IV bolus: 1–10 mg, give over 3–5 min
  IV infusion: dilute with 55 ml glucose 5%; give over 60 min. Solution should be freshly prepared and protected from light
  Not for IM injection

Maximum dose: 40 mg in 24 h

How not to use vitamin K
Do not give by rapid IV bolus
Do not give IM injections in patients with abnormal clotting
Not for the reversal of heparin

Adverse effects
Hypersensitivity

Cautions
Onset of action slow (use FFP if rapid effect needed)

VORICONAZOLE (Vfend)

Voriconazole is a broad-spectrum, triazole antifungal agent that is used mainly to treat invasive aspergillosis. In contrast to echinocandins, it has an oral form as well as an IV formulation, which makes it suitable for long-term therapy. However, it can cause hepatoxicity, which requires cessation of therapy. It also interacts significantly with drugs commonly used in the ICU, which can complicate treatment.

Uses
Treatment of invasive aspergillosis; serious infections caused by *Scedosporium* spp., *Fusarium* spp., or invasive fluconazole-resistant *Candida* spp. (including *C. krusei*).

Contraindications
Acute porphyria

Administration
IV: 6 mg/kg every 12 hours for 2 doses, then 4 mg/kg every 12 hours (reduced to 3 mg/kg every 12 hours if not tolerated) for max. 6 months. Reconstitute each vial with 19 ml WFI to make a 200 mg/20 ml solution. Add dose to sodium chloride 0.9% or glucose 5% bag, the final solution should be 2–5 mg/ml. Administer over 2 hours

PO/NG: 40 kg, 400 mg 12 hourly for 2 doses then 200 mg 12 hourly, increased if necessary to 300 mg 12 hourly

<40 kg, 200 mg 12 hourly for 2 doses then 100 mg 12 hourly, increased if necessary to 150 mg 12 hourly. Available as 200 mg, 50 mg tabs and 250 mg/5 ml oral suspension. Take oral dose 1 hour before or an hour after meals (or turn ng feed off for 1 hour before and after dosing)

Adverse effects
Jaundice
Oedema, hypotension
Chest pain, respiratory distress syndrome
Headache, dizziness, asthenia, anxiety, depression
Confusion, agitation, hallucinations, paraesthesia, tremor
Hypoglycaemia, haematuria, blood disorders
Acute renal failure, hypokalaemia, visual disturbances

Cautions
Cardiomyopathy, bradycardia
Symptomatic arrhythmias, history of QT prolongation, concomitant use with other drugs that prolong QT interval
Those at risk of pancreatitis

Key interactions
Voriconazole inhibits the activity of cytochrome P450 and increases levels of the following:

alfenatnil, artemether/lumefantrine, ciclosporin, clopidogrel, warfarin, diazepam, dronedarone (avoid), efavirenz, fentanyl, methadone, midazolam, oxycodone, phenytoin, quetiapine, rifabutin, sirolimus, tacrolimus, tretinoin

Voriconazole is also metabolised by cytochrome P450; the following drugs affect voriconazole levels:

carbamazepine, efavirenz, phenobarbital (avoid), phenytoin, rifabutin, rifampicin (avoid), ritonavir (avoid), telaprevir

Organ failure
Renal: PO/NG no dose adjustment needed
IV: if CC <50 ml/min, the IV vehicle SBECD accumulates. If PO/NG not suitable, then continue with IV but assess risk–benefit ratio; SBECD is removed by HD

Liver: mild-moderate hepatic cirrhosis use usual initial dose then halve subsequent doses. No information available for severe hepatic cirrhosis; manufacturer advises use only if potential benefit outweighs risk

ZINC

Zinc is an essential constituent of many enzymes. Deficiencies in zinc may result in poor wound healing. Zinc deficiency can occur in patients on inadequate diets, in malabsorption, with increased catabolism due to trauma, burns and protein-losing conditions, and during TPN.

Hypoproteinaemia spuriously lowers plasma zinc levels.

Normal range: 12–23 µmol/l

Uses
Zinc deficiency
As an antioxidant (p. 288)

Administration
- Orally: zinc sulphate effervescent tablet 125 mg dissolved in water, 1–3 times daily after food
- IV: 1 mmol zinc sulphate diluted in 250 ml glucose 5% or sodium chloride 0.9%, given over 2 hours

Available as 1 mmol zinc sulphate in 10 ml vial

Adverse effects
Abdominal pains
Dyspepsia

ROUTES OF ADMINISTRATION

Intravenous
This is the most common route employed in the critically ill. It is reliable, having no problems of absorption, avoids first-pass metabolism and has a rapid onset of action. Its disadvantages include the increased risk of serious side-effects and the possibility of phlebitis or tissue necrosis if extravasation occurs.

Intramuscular
The need for frequent, painful injections, the presence of a coagulopathy (risk the development of a haematoma, which may become infected) and the lack of muscle bulk often seen in the critically ill means that this route is seldom used in the critically ill. Furthermore, variable absorption because of changes in cardiac output and blood flow to muscles, posture and site of injection makes absorption unpredictable.

Subcutaneous
Rarely used, except for low molecular weight heparin when used for prophylaxis against DVT. Absorption is variable and unreliable.

Oral
In the critically ill this route includes administrations via NG, NJ, PEG, PEJ or surgical jejunostomy feeding tubes. Medications given via these enteral feeding tubes should be liquid or finely crushed, dissolved in water. Rinsing should take place before and after feed or medication has been administered, using 20–30 ml WFI. In the seriously ill patient this route is not commonly used to give drugs. Note than some liquid preparations contain sorbitol, which has a laxative effect at daily doses >15 g. An example of this is baclofen, where the Lioresal liquid preparation contains 2.75 g/5 ml of sorbitol, so a dose of 20 mg 6 hourly would deliver 44 g of sorbitol. In these cases it is preferable to crush tablets than to administer liquid preparations. The effect of pain and its treatment with opioids, variations in splanchnic blood flow and changes in intestinal transit times – as well as variability in hepatic function, make it an unpredictable and unreliable way of giving drugs.

Buccal and sublingual
Avoids the problem of oral absorption and first-pass metabolism, and it has a rapid onset time. It has been used for GTN, buprenorphine and nifedipine.

Rectal

Avoids the problems of oral absorption. Absorption may be variable and unpredictable. It depends on absorption from the rectum and from the anal canal. Drugs absorbed from the rectum (superior haemorrhoidal vein) are subject to hepatic metabolism; those from the anal canal enter the systemic circulation directly. Levothyroxine tablets can be used rectally (unlicensed) when the oral route is unavailable.

Tracheobronchial

Useful for drugs acting directly on the lungs: β_2-agonists, anticholinergics and corticosteroids. It offers the advantage of a rapid onset of action and a low risk of systemic side effects.

LOADING DOSE

An initial loading dose is given quickly to increase the plasma concentration of a drug to the desired steady-state concentration. This is particularly important for drugs with long half-lives (amiodarone, digoxin). It normally takes five half-lives to reach steady-state if the usual doses are given at the recommended interval. Thus, steady-state may not be reached for many days. There are two points worth noting:

- For IV bolus administration, the plasma concentration of a drug after a loading dose can be considerably higher than that desired, resulting in toxicity, albeit transiently. This is important for drugs with a low therapeutic index (digoxin, theophylline). To prevent excessive drug concentrations, slow IV administration of these drugs is recommended.
- For drugs that are excreted by the kidneys unchanged (gentamicin, digoxin) reduction of the maintenance dose is needed to prevent accumulation. No reduction in the loading dose is needed.

DRUG METABOLISM

Most drugs are lipid-soluble and, therefore, cannot be excreted unchanged in the urine or bile. Water-soluble drugs such as the aminoglycosides and digoxin are excreted unchanged by the kidneys. The liver is the major site of drug metabolism. The main purpose of drug metabolism is to make the drug more water-soluble so that it can be excreted. Metabolism can be divided into two types:

- Phase 1 reactions are simple chemical reactions including oxidation, reduction, hydroxylation and acetylation.
- Phase 2 reactions are conjugations with glucuronide, sulphate or glycine. Many of the reactions are catalysed by groups of enzyme systems.

ENZYME SYSTEMS

These enzyme systems are capable of being induced or inhibited. Enzyme induction usually takes place over several days; induction of enzymes by a drug leads not only to an increase in its own metabolic degradation, but also often that of other drugs. This usually leads to a decrease in effect of the drug, unless the metabolite is active or toxic. Conversely, inhibition of the enzyme systems will lead to an increased effect. Inhibition of enzymes is quick, usually needing only one or two doses of the drug. Below are examples of enzyme inducers and inhibitors:

Inducers	Inhibitors
Barbiturates	Amiodarone
Carbamazepine	Cimetidine
Ethanol (chronic)	Ciprofloxacin
Inhalational anaesthetics	Ethanol (acute)
Griseofulvin	Etomidate
Phenytoin	Erythromycin
Primidone	Fluconazole
Rifampicin	Ketoconazole
	Metronidazole

DRUG EXCRETION

Almost all drugs and/or their metabolites (with the exception of the inhalational anaesthetics) are eventually eliminated from the body in urine or in bile. Compounds with a low molecular weight are excreted in the urine. By contrast, compounds with a high molecular weight are eliminated in the bile. This route plays an important part in the elimination of penicillins, pancuronium and vecuronium.

DRUG TOLERANCE

Tolerance to a drug will over time diminish its effectiveness. Tolerance to the effects of opioids is thought to be a result of a change in the receptors. Other receptors will become less sensitive with a reduction in their number over time when stimulated with large amounts of drug or endogenous agonist, for example catecholamines. Tolerance to the organic nitrates may be the result of the reduced metabolism of these drugs to the active molecule, nitric oxide, as a result of a depletion within blood vessels of compounds containing the sulphydryl group. Acetylcysteine, a sulphydryl group donor, is occasionally used to prevent nitrate tolerance.

DRUG INTERACTIONS

Two or more drugs given at the same time may exert their effects independently or may interact. The potential for interaction increases the greater the number of drugs employed. Most patients admitted to an intensive care unit will be on more than one drug.

Drugs interactions can be grouped into three principal subdivisions: pharmacokinetic, pharmacodynamic and pharmaceutical.

- Pharmacokinetic interactions are those that include transport to and from the receptor site and consist of absorption, distribution, metabolism and excretion.
- Pharmacodynamic interactions occur between drugs which have similar or antagonistic pharmacological effects or side-effects. This may be due to competition at receptor sites or can occur between drugs acting on the same physiological system. They are usually predictable from a knowledge of the pharmacology of the interacting drugs.
- Pharmaceutical interactions are physical, and chemical incompatibilities may result in loss of potency, increase in toxicity or other adverse effects. The solutions may become opalescent or precipitation may occur, but in many instances there is no visual indication of incompatibility. Precipitation reactions may occur as a result of pH, concentration changes or 'salting-out' effects.

THERAPEUTIC DRUG MONITORING

The serum drug concentration should never be interpreted in isolation, and the patient's clinical condition must be considered. The sample must be taken at the correct time in relation to dosage interval.

Phenytoin

Phenytoin has a low therapeutic index and a narrow target range. Although the average daily dose is 300 mg, the dose needed for a concentration in the target range varies from 100 to 700 mg/day. Because phenytoin has non-linear (zero-order) kinetics, small increases in dose can result in greater increases in blood level.

Aminoglycosides

Gentamicin, tobramycin, netilmicin and amikacin are antibiotics with a low therapeutic index. After starting treatment, measurements should be made before and after the third to fifth dose in those with normal renal function, and earlier in those with abnormal renal function. Levels should be repeated, if the dose requires adjustment, after another 2 doses. If renal function is stable and the dose correct, a further check should be made every 3 days, but more frequently in those patients whose renal function is changing rapidly. It is often necessary to adjust both the dose and the dose interval to ensure that both peak and trough concentrations remain within the target ranges. In spite of careful monitoring, the risk of toxicity increases with the duration of treatment and the concurrent use of loop diuretics.

Vancomycin

This glycopeptide antibiotic is highly ototoxic and nephrotoxic. Monitoring of serum concentrations is essential, especially in the presence of renal impairment.

Theophylline

Individual variation in theophylline metabolism is considerable and the drug has a low therapeutic index. Concurrent treatment with cimetidine, erythromycin and certain 4-quinolones (ciprofloxacin, norfloxacin) can result in toxicity due to enzyme inhibition of theophylline metabolism.

Digoxin

In the management of AF, the drug response (ventricular rate) can be assessed directly. Monitoring may be indicated if renal function should deteriorate and other drugs (amiodarone and verapamil) are used concurrently. The slow absorption and distribution of the drug means that the sample should be taken at least 6 h after the oral dose is given. For IV administration, sampling time is not critical.

TARGET RANGE OF CONCENTRATION

Drug	Sampling time(s) after dose	Threshold for therapeutic effect	Threshold for toxic effect
Teicoplanin	Trough: pre-dose	Trough: >10 mg/l Severe infections require >20 mg/l	None defined
Gentamicin Tobramycin Netilmicin	Peak: 1 hour after bolus or at end of infusion Trough: pre-dose	Peak: 10 mg/l	Trough: 2 mg/l
Vancomycin	Peak: 2 h after end of infusion Trough: pre-dose	Trough: 5–10 mg/l May need 15–20 mg/l for MRSA	Peak >30– 40 mg/l
Phenytoin	Trough: pre-dose	10 mg/l (40 µmol/l)	20 mg/l (80 µmol/l)
Theophylline	Trough: pre-dose	10 mg/l (55 µmol/l)	20 mg/l (110 µmol/l)
Digoxin	At least 6 h	0.8 µg/l (1 nmol/l)	Typically >3 µg/l (3.8 nmol/l), but may be lower dependent on plasma electrolytes, thyroid function, PaO_2

The target range lies between the lowest effective concentration and the highest safe concentration. Efficacy is best reflected by the peak level, and safety (toxicity) is best reflected by the trough level (except for vancomycin). The dosage may be manipulated by altering the dosage interval or the dose or both. If the pre–dose value is greater than the trough, increasing the dosage interval is appropriate. If the post–dose value is greater than the peak, dose reduction would be appropriate.

PHARMACOLOGY IN THE CRITICALLY ILL

In the critically ill patient, changes of function in the liver, kidneys and other organs may result in alterations in drug effect and elimination. These changes may not be constant in the critically ill patient, but may improve or worsen as the patient's condition changes. In addition, these changes will affect not only the drugs themselves but also their metabolites, many of which may be active.

Hepatic disease

Hepatic disease may alter the response to drugs, in several ways:

- Impairment of liver function slows elimination of drugs, resulting in prolongation of action and accumulation of the drug or its metabolites.
- With hypoproteinaemia there is decreased protein binding of some drugs. This increases the amount of free (active) drug.
- Bilirubin competes with many drugs for the binding sites on serum albumin. This also increases the amount of free drug.
- Reduced hepatic synthesis of clotting factors increases the sensitivity to warfarin.
- Hepatic encephalopathy may be precipitated by all sedative drugs, opioids and diuretics that produce hypokalaemia (thiazides and loop diuretics).
- Fluid overload may be exacerbated by drugs that cause fluid retention, e.g. NSAID and corticosteroids.
- Renal function may be depressed. It follows that drugs having a major renal route of elimination may be affected in liver disease, because of the secondary development of functional renal impairment.
- Hepatotoxic drugs should be avoided.

Renal impairment

Impairment of renal function may result in failure to excrete a drug or its metabolites. The degree of renal impairment can be measured using creatinine clearance, which requires 24-hour urine collection. It can be estimated by calculation using serum creatinine (see Appendix A). Most of the published evidence on dosing in renal failure is based on the Cockcroft–Gault equation. Serum creatinine depends on age, sex and muscle mass. The elderly patients and the critically ill may have creatinine clearances <50 ml/min but, because of reduced muscle mass, increased serum creatinine may appear 'normal'. The eGFR is increasingly reported. It should be recognised that it is normalised to a standardised body surface area of 1.73 m^2. The eGFR should not be used to calculate drug doses for those at high or low body mass, nor for drugs with a low therapeutic index, unless it is first corrected to the actual GFR with the following equation:

$$\text{Actual GFR} = \text{eGFR} \times \text{Body surface area}/1.73$$

When the creatinine clearance is >30 ml/min, it is seldom necessary to modify normal doses, except for certain antibiotics and cardiovascular drugs which are excreted unchanged by the kidneys. There is no need to decrease the initial or loading dose. Maintenance doses are adjusted by either lengthening the interval between doses or by reducing the size of individual doses, or a combination of both. Therapeutic drug monitoring, when available, is an invaluable guide to therapy.

Haemofiltration or dialysis does not usually replace the normal excretory function of the kidneys. A reduction in dose may be needed for drug eliminated by the kidneys.

Nephrotoxic drugs should, if possible, be avoided. These include furosemide, thiazides, sulphonamides, penicillins, aminoglycosides and rifampicin.

Cardiac failure

Drug absorption may be impaired because of GI mucosal congestion. Dosages of drugs that are mainly metabolised by the liver or mainly excreted by the kidneys may need to be modified. This is because of impaired drug delivery to the liver, which delays metabolism, and impaired renal function leading to delayed elimination.

CARDIOPULMONARY RESUSCITATION

Adult Advanced Life Support Algorithm (The Resuscitation Council (UK) Guidelines 2010). Reproduced with the kind permission of the Resuscitation Council (UK)

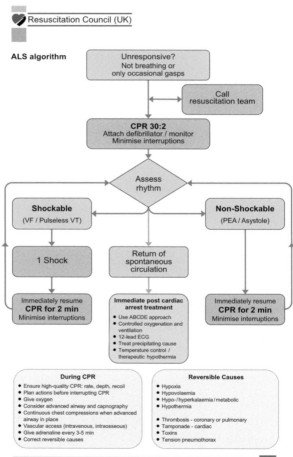

Resuscitation Council (UK)

ALS algorithm

Unresponsive?
Not breathing or
only occasional gasps

Call resuscitation team

CPR 30:2
Attach defibrillator / monitor
Minimise interruptions

Assess rhythm

Shockable
(VF / Pulseless VT)

Non-Shockable
(PEA / Asystole)

1 Shock

Return of spontaneous circulation

Immediately resume
CPR for 2 min
Minimise interruptions

Immediate post cardiac arrest treatment
- Use ABCDE approach
- Controlled oxygenation and ventilation
- 12-lead ECG
- Treat precipitating cause
- Temperature control / therapeutic hypothermia

Immediately resume
CPR for 2 min
Minimise interruptions

During CPR
- Ensure high-quality CPR: rate, depth, recoil
- Plan actions before interrupting CPR
- Give oxygen
- Consider advanced airway and capnography
- Continuous chest compressions when advanced airway in place
- Vascular access (intravenous, intraosseous)
- Give adrenaline every 3-5 min
- Correct reversible causes

Reversible Causes
- Hypoxia
- Hypovolaemia
- Hypo-/hyperkalaemia/metabolic
- Hypothermia

- Thrombosis - coronary or pulmonary
- Tamponade - cardiac
- Toxins
- Tension pneumothorax

Summary of main changes

Adult advanced life support

There are several changes to the ALS guidelines and, for simplicity, these are grouped by topic.

Defibrillation

- There is increased emphasis on the importance of minimal interruption in high-quality chest compressions throughout any ALS intervention: chest compressions are paused briefly only to enable specific planned interventions.

- The recommendation for a specified period of CPR before out-of-hospital defibrillation following cardiac arrest unwitnessed by the EMS has been removed.

- Chest compressions are now continued while a defibrillator is charged – this will minimise the preshock pause.

- The role of the **precordial thump is de-emphasised**.

- There is inclusion of the use of up to three quick successive (stacked) shocks for ventricular fibrillation/pulseless ventricular tachycardia (VF/VT) occurring in the cardiac catheterisation laboratory or in the immediate postoperative period following cardiac surgery.

Drugs

- **Delivery of drugs via a tracheal tube is no longer recommended** – if intravenous (IV) access cannot be achieved, give drugs by the intraosseous **(IO) route**.

- When treating VF/VT cardiac arrest, adrenaline 1 mg is given once chest compressions have restarted after the third shock and then every 3–5 min (during alternate cycles of CPR). Amiodarone 300 mg is also given after the third shock.

- **Atropine is no longer recommended for routine use in asystole or pulseless electrical activity**.

Airway

- There is reduced emphasis on early tracheal intubation unless achieved by highly skilled individuals with minimal interruption to chest compressions.

- There is increased emphasis on the use of capnography to confirm and continually monitor tracheal tube placement and quality of CPR and to provide an early indication of return of spontaneous circulation (ROSC).

Post–resuscitation care

- There is recognition of the potential harm caused by hyperoxaemia after ROSC is achieved: once ROSC has been established and the oxygen saturation of arterial blood (SaO_2) can be monitored reliably (by pulse oximetry and/or arterial blood gas analysis), inspired oxygen is titrated to achieve a SaO_2 of 94%–98%.

- There is much greater detail and emphasis on the treatment of the postcardiac-arrest syndrome.

- There is recognition that implementation of a comprehensive, structured postresuscitation treatment protocol may improve survival in cardiac arrest victims after ROSC.

- There is increased emphasis on the use of primary percutaneous coronary intervention in appropriate but comatose patients with sustained ROSC after cardiac arrest.

- There is revision of the recommendation for glucose control: in adults with sustained ROSC after cardiac arrest, blood glucose values >10 mmol/1 should be treated but hypoglycaemia must be avoided.

- Use of therapeutic hypothermia to include comatose survivors of cardiac arrest associated initially with non-shockable rhythms as well as shockable rhythms. The lower level of evidence for use after cardiac arrest from non-shockable rhythms is acknowledged.

- There is recognition that many of the accepted predictors of poor outcome in comatose survivors of cardiac arrest are unreliable, especially if the patient has been treated with therapeutic hypothermia.

DRUGS IN ADVANCED LIFE SUPPORT

In VF/pulseless VT arrest, the administration of drugs should not delay DC shocks. Defibrillation is still the only intervention capable of restoring a spontaneous circulation. In EMD or PEA (pulseless electrical activity), the search for specific and correctable causes (4 Hs and 4 Ts) is of prime importance. If no evidence exists for any specific cause CPR should be continued, with the use of adrenaline every 3–5 min.

Adrenaline (epinephrine) 1 mg (10 ml 1 in 10 000/1 ml 1 in 1000)

Adrenaline has both alpha and beta effects. The alpha effect increases perfusion pressure and thus myocardial and cerebral blood flow. The beta-1 effect helps to maintain cardiac output after spontaneous heart action has been restored.

• VF/VT

When treating VF/VT cardiac arrest, adrenaline 1 mg is given once chest compressions have restarted after the third shock and then every 3–5 min (during alternate cycles of CPR).

• PEA/asystole

Give adrenaline 1 mg IV as soon as IV access is achieved and repeat every 3–5 min.

Amiodarone 300 mg IV

If VF/VT persists after the third shock, give amiodarone 300 mg as an IV bolus. A further 150 mg may be given for recurrent or refractory VF/VT, followed by an IV infusion of 900 mg over 24 h.

Magnesium 8 mmol IV (4 ml 50% solution)

Give magnesium 8 mmol for refractory VF if there is any suspicion of hypomagnesaemia (e.g. patients on potassium-losing diuretics). Other indications are:

• ventricular tachyarrhythmias in the presence of hypomagnesaemia
• torsade de pointes
• digoxin toxicity

Calcium chloride 1 g IV (10 ml 10% solution)

Adequate levels of ionised calcium are necessary for effective cardiovascular function. Ionised calcium concentrations decrease during prolonged (>7.5 min) cardiac arrest. The chloride salt is preferred to the gluconate salt, as it does not require hepatic metabolism to release the calcium ion. 10 ml 10% calcium chloride provides 6.8 mmol Ca^{2+} (10 ml 10% calcium gluconate provides only 2.25 mmol Ca^{2+}).

Caution: calcium overload is thought to play an important role in ischaemic and reperfusion cell injury. It may also be implicated in coronary artery spasm. Excessive doses should not be used.

Calcium chloride is indicated in:

- hypocalcaemia
- hyperkalaemia
- calcium–channel antagonist overdose
- magnesium overdose

Sodium bicarbonate 50 mmol (50 ml 8.4% solution)

Routine use of sodium bicarbonate during cardiac arrest is not recommended.

Give 50 mmol of sodium bicarbonate if cardiac arrest is associated with hyperkalaemia or tricyclic antidepressant overdose. Repeat the dose according to the results of repeated blood gas analysis. Several problems are associated with its use:

(i) CO_2 released passes across the cell membrane and increases intracellular pH.

(ii) The development of an iatrogenic extracellular alkalosis may be even less favourable than acidosis.

(iii) It may induce hyperosmolarity, causing a decrease in aortic diastolic pressure and therefore a decrease in coronary perfusion pressure.

Do not let sodium bicarbonate come into contact with catecholamines (inactivates) or calcium salts (precipitates).

Tracheobronchial route for drugs

Delivery of drugs via a tracheal tube is no longer recommended – if intravenous (IV) access cannot be achieved, give drugs by the **intraosseous (IO) route**.

MANAGEMENT OF ACUTE MAJOR ANAPHYLAXIS

- **Immediate therapy**

Stop giving the suspect drug

Maintain airway, give 100% oxygen

Adrenaline 50–100 µg (0.5–1.0 ml 1:10 000) IV

Further 100 µg bolus PRN for hypotension and bronchospasm

Crystalloid 500–1000 ml rapidly

- **Secondary management**

For adrenaline-resistant bronchospasm:

salbutamol 250 µg IV loading dose

5–20 µg/min maintenance

dilute 5 mg in 500 ml glucose 5% or sodium chloride 0.9% (10 µg/ml)

or

aminophylline 5 mg/kg

in 500 ml sodium chloride 0.9%, IV infusion over 5 hours

To prevent further deterioration:

hydrocortisone 200 mg IV

and

chlorphenamine 20 mg IV

dilute with 10 ml sodium chloride 0.9% or WFI given over 1–2 min

- **Investigation**

Plasma tryptase: contact the biochemistry lab first. Take 2 ml blood in an EDTA tube at the following times: as soon as possible (within 1 h), at 3 hours and at 24 hours (as control). The samples should be sent *immediately* to the lab for the plasma to be separated and frozen at 20°C.

In the UK, when all the samples have been collected, they will be sent to: Department of Immunology, Northern General Hospital, Herries Road, Sheffield, S5 7AU; Telephone: 0114 2715552.

Assay for urinary methyl histamine is no longer available.

MANAGEMENT OF SEVERE HYPERKALAEMIA

Criteria for treatment:

- K^+ >6.5 mmol/l
- ECG changes (peaked T, wide QRS)
- Severe weakness

Calcium chloride 10–20 ml 10% IV over 5–10 min

This increases the cell depolarisation threshold and reduces myocardial irritability. It results in improvement in ECG changes within seconds, but because the K^+ levels are not altered, the effect lasts only about 30 min.

Soluble insulin 10 units with 125 ml glucose 20% or 250 ml glucose 10%

Given IV over 30–60 min. Begins lowering serum K^+ in 2–5 min and the effect lasting 1–2 hours. Monitor blood glucose.

Sodium bicarbonate 50 mmol (50 ml 8.4%)

By correcting the acidosis its effect again is only transient. Beware in patients with fluid overload.

Calcium resonium 15 g PO or 30 g as retention enema, 8 hourly

This will draw the K^+ from the gut and remove K^+ from the body. Oral lactulose 20 ml 8 hourly may induce a mild diarrhoea, which helps to remove K^+ and also avoids constipation when resins are used.

Haemofiltration/dialysis

Indicated if plasma K^+ persistently $\uparrow$, acidosis, uraemia or serious fluid overload is already present.

MANAGEMENT OF MALIGNANT HYPERTHERMIA

Clinical features

- Jaw spasm immediately after suxamethonium
- Generalised muscle rigidity
- Unexplained tachycardia, tachypnoea, sweating and cyanosis
- Increase in ETCO$_2$
- Rapid increase in body temperature (>4°C/h)

Management

- Inform surgical team and send for experienced help
- Elective surgery: abandon procedure, monitor and treat
- Emergency surgery: finish as soon as possible, switch to 'safe agents', monitor and treat
- Stop all inhalational anaesthetics
- Change to vapour-free anaesthetic machine and hyperventilate with 100% O$_2$ at 2–3 times predicted minute volume
- Give dantrolene 1 mg/kg IV
  Response to dantrolene should begin to occur in minutes (decreased muscle tone, heart rate and temperature); if not, repeat every 5 min, up to a total of 10 mg/kg
- Give sodium bicarbonate 100 ml 8.4% IV
  Further doses guided by arterial blood gas
- Correct hyperkalaemia with 50 ml glucose 50% and 10 units insulin over 30 min
- Correct cardiac arrhythmias according to their nature (usually respond to correction of acidosis, hypercarbia and hyperkalaemia)
- Start active cooling
  Refrigerated sodium chloride 0.9% IV 1–2 l initially (avoid Hartmann's solution because of its potassium content)
  Surface cooling: ice packs and fans (may be ineffective due to peripheral vasoconstriction)
  Lavage of peritoneal and gastric cavities with refrigerated sodium chloride 0.9%
- Maintain urine output with:
  IV fluids
  Mannitol
  Furosemide

Monitoring and investigations

ECG, BP and capnography (if not already)
Oesophageal or rectal temperature: core temperature
Urinary catheter: send urine for myoglobin and measure urine output
Arterial line: arterial gas analysis, U&E and creatine phosphokinase
Central venous line: CVP and IV fluids
Fluid balance chart: sweating loss to be accounted for

After the crisis
Admit to ICU for at least 24 h (crisis can recur)
Monitor potassium, creatine phosphokinase, myoglobinuria,
temperature, renal failure and clotting status
May need to repeat dantrolene (half-life only 5 h)
Investigate patient and family for susceptibility

Triggering agents
Suxamethonium
All potent inhalational anaesthetic agents

Safe drug
All benzodiazepines
Thiopentone, propofol
All non-depolarising muscle relaxants
All opioids
Nitrous oxide
All local anaesthetic agents
Neostigmine, atropine, glycopyrrolate
Droperidol, metoclopramide

SEDATION, ANALGESIA AND NEUROMUSCULAR BLOCKADE

The ideal level of sedation should leave a patient lightly asleep but easily roused. Opioids, in combination with a benzodiazepine or propofol, are currently the most frequently used agents for sedation, although benzodiazepines are associated with delirium and are increasingly avoided.

The most common indication for the therapeutic use of opioids is to provide analgesia. They are also able to elevate mood and suppress the cough reflex. This antitussive effect is a useful adjunct to their analgesic effects in patients who need to tolerate a tracheal tube.

Propofol has achieved widespread popularity for sedation. It is easily titrated to achieve the desired level of sedation and its effects end rapidly when the infusion is stopped, even after several days of use. Propofol is ideal for short periods of sedation on the ICU, and during weaning when longer-acting agents are being eliminated. Some clinicians recommend propofol for long-term sedation.

Currently, new sedative and analgesic drugs are designed to be short-acting. This means that they usually have to be given by continuous IV infusion. The increased cost of these drugs may be justifiable if they give better control and more predictable analgesia and sedation, and allow quicker weaning from ventilatory support.

Midazolam, the shortest acting of all the benzodiazepines, is the most widely used of the benzodiazepines. It can be given either by infusion or intermittent bolus doses.

NSAIDS have an opioid-sparing effect and are of particular benefit for the relief of pain from bones and joints, as well as the general aches and pains associated with prolonged immobilisation. However, their use in the critically ill is significantly limited by their side-effects, which include reduced platelet aggregation, gastrointestinal haemorrhage and deterioration in renal function.

Antidepressants may be useful in patients recovering from a prolonged period of critical illness. At this time depression and sleep disturbances are common. The use of amitriptyline is well established and relatively safe, but it has a higher incidence of antimuscarinic or cardiac side-effects than the newer agents. The beneficial effect may not be apparent until 2–4 weeks after starting the drug, so any benefits may not be seen on the ICU. Cardiovascular effects, in particular arrhythmias, have not proved to be a problem. Whether the newer SSRIs (e.g. fluoxetine) will have any advantages in the critically ill remains to be proved.

Clomethiazole has sedative and anticonvulsant properties. It is usually reserved for patients with an alcohol problem for treatment in hospital. It is not safe to discharge patients with clomethiazole.

Chlordiazepoxide is widely used as an alternative for alcohol withdrawal, see section on p. 274.

Muscle relaxants are neither analgesic nor sedative agents and, therefore, should not be used without ensuring that the patient is both pain-free and unaware. Their use has declined since the introduction of synchronised modes of ventilation and more sophisticated electronic control mechanisms. Their use is also associated with critical illness polyneuropathy. Suxamethonium, atracurium and vecuronium are presently the most commonly used agents, although pancuronium is still used in certain ICUs. Their use should be restricted to certain specific indications:

- tracheal intubation
- facilitation of procedures, e.g. tracheostomy
- ARDS, where oxygenation is critical and there is risk of barotrauma
- management of neurosurgical or head injured patients where coughing or straining on the tracheal tube increases ICP
- to stop the spasm of tetanus

Regular monitoring with a peripheral nerve stimulator is desirable; ablation of more than 3 twitches of the train-of-four is very rarely necessary.

Delirium

Delirium is increasingly recognised as an outward manifestation of brain dysfunction. Delirium in hospital is a strong risk factor for increased mortality in hospital and for 11 months after discharge. It is common in the ICU and occurs as hypoactive, mixed or hyperactive manifestation. The CAM-ICU assessment method is commonly used to monitor for delirium. There are many non-drug potential causes, including noise, lack of glasses, language, poor nutrition, insomnia, dehydration, infection, dementia, depression, pain, hypoxia and use of physical restraints.

Drugs that can contribute to delirium.

	Examples
Analgesics	Opioids, NSAIDs
Hypnotics	Benzodiazepines, Chloral hydrate, Thiopental
Anticholinergics	Atropine, Hyoscine
Antihistamines	Chlorpheniramine, Promethazine
Anticonvulsants	Phenytoin, Carbamazepine, Valproic acid
Anti-Parkinson's agents	Levodopa, Amantadine
H_2 blockers	Ranitidine
Antibiotics	Penicillin
Cardiac drugs	Beta-blockers, Clonidine, Digoxin, Methyldopa
Corticosteroids	Dexamethasone, Hydrocortisone, Prednisolone
Anti-emetics	Metoclopramide, Prochlorperezine
Anti-depressants	Amitryptyline, Paroxetine
Cardiovascular drugs	Digoxin, Atenolol, Dopamine, Lidocaine
Miscellaneous	Frusemide, Isoflurane, Substance withdrawal

Treatment of ICU delirium

Identification of the potential cause of delirium will determine the treatment. Efforts should be made to promote night-time sleep by altering the environment (reducing noise, light, etc.). Haloperidol is the mainstay of drug treatment. Although some brands are not licensed for IV use in the UK, IV therapy is standard practice. The main side effects to monitor for are *torsades de pointes*, extrapyramidal side effects and risk of developing neuroleptic malignant syndrome. In such cases olanzapine, quetiapine or risperidone are alternatives, although these are still a caution in *torsades de pointes* and are not necessarily safe. Rivastigmine should not be used in delirious patients. Benzodiazepines remain the treatment of choice for alcohol withdrawal. No pharmacological therapy has been shown to prevent delirium.

Morphine IM injection to oral tramadol:

40 mg morphine daily by injection: conversion factor = × 2

= 40 × 2 = 80 mg oral morphine daily

Tramadol: conversion factor: ÷ 0.2

= 80 ÷ 0.2 = 400 mg tramadol total daily dose, i.e. 100 mg 6 hourly

Remember:

When converting a patient from regular oral morphine (immediate release) to MST (modified release):
Add up the total amount of morphine administered in 24 hours
Halve this amount to give a twice daily (bd) MST dose
e.g. 10 mg qds immediate release morphine = 40 mg in 24 hours = 20 mg bd MST

Transdermal fentanyl

The initial fentanyl patch dose should be based on the patient's previous opioid history, including the degree of opioid tolerance, if any. The lowest dose 25 μg/hour should be initiated in strong-opioid–naïve patients. In opioid-tolerant patients, the initial dose of fentanyl should be based on the previous 24-hour opioid analgesic requirement. A recommended conversion scheme from oral morphine is given below:

Oral 24–hour morphine (mg/day)	Transdermal fentanyl dose (μg/h)
<135	25
135–224	50
225–314	75
315–404	100
405–494	125
495–584	150
585–674	175
675–764	200
765–854	225
855–944	250
945–1034	275
1035–1124	300

For both strong opioid-naïve and opioid-tolerant patients the initial evaluation of the analgesic effect of the transdermal fentanyl should not be made before the patch has been worn for 24 hours, due to gradual increase in serum fentanyl concentrations up to this time. Previous analgesic therapy should therefore be phased out gradually from the time of the first patch application until analgesic efficacy with fentanyl is attained.

Remember:
Fentanyl levels fall gradually once the patch is removed, taking up to 17 hours or more for the fentanyl serum concentration to decrease by 50%.

A PRACTICAL APPROACH TO SEDATION AND ANALGESIA

SHORT NOTES

MANAGEMENT OF STATUS EPILEPTICUS

Status epilepticus is defined as continuous seizure activity lasting >30 min or more than two discrete seizures, between which the patient does not recover consciousness. About 50% of patients have known epilepsy, and status may be secondary to poor drug compliance with anticonvulsant therapy, a change in anticonvulsant therapy or alcohol withdrawal. Other causes of status epilepticus are listed below.

History of epilepsy

- Poor compliance
- Recent change in medication
- Drug interactions
- Withdrawal of the effects of alcohol
- Pseudostatus

No history of epilepsy

- Intracranial tumour/abscess
- Intracranial haemorrhage
- Stroke
- Head injury or surgery
- Infection – meningitis, encephalitis
- Febrile convulsions in children
- Metabolic abnormalities – hypoglycaemia, hypocalcaemia, hyponatraemia, hypomagnesaemia, hypoxia
- Drug toxicity
- Drug or alcohol withdrawal
- Use of antagonists in mixed drug overdoses

Status epilepticus is divided into four stages. There is usually a preceding period of increasing seizures – **the premonitory stage**, which can be treated with a benzodiazepine such as clobazam 10 mg. Early treatment at this stage may prevent the development of the next stage. **Early status epilepticus** can usually be terminated by an IV bolus of lorazepam 4 mg, repeated after 10 min if no response. If there is no response to benzodiazepine therapy after 30 min, **established status epilepticus** has developed and either phenobarbital, phenytoin or fosphenytoin should be given. If a patient is in **refractory status epilepticus** (when seizure activity has lasted 1 h and there has been no response to prior therapy), the patient should be transferred to ICU and given a general anaesthetic to abolish electrographic seizure activity and prevent further cerebral damage.

The initial management of status epilepticus is directed at supporting vital functions. This is the same as that for any medical emergency, including assessment of airways, breathing and circulation.

IV **lorazepam** may now be the preferred first-line drug for stopping status epilepticus. Lorazepam carries a lower risk of cardiorespiratory depression (respiratory arrest, hypotension) than **diazepam** as it is less lipid-soluble. Lorazepam also has a longer duration of anticonvulsant activity compared with diazepam (6–12 h versus 15–30 min after a single bolus). If IV access cannot be obtained diazepam may be given rectally (Stesolid). It takes up to 10 min to work. The duration of action of diazepam in the brain is short (15–30 min) because of rapid redistribution. This means that, although a diazepam bolus is effective at stopping a fit, it will not prevent further fits.

If there is no response to benzodiazepine treatment after 30 min, either **phenobarbital**, **phenytoin** or **fosphenytoin** should be given. Fosphenytoin is a water-soluble phosphate ester of phenytoin that is converted rapidly after IV administration to phenytoin by endogenous phosphatases. An advantage of IV fosphenytoin is that it can be given up to three times faster than phenytoin without significant cardiovascular side-effects (hypotension, arrhythmias). It can also be given IM, unlike phenytoin. Fosphenytoin may some day replace phenytoin. Patients with known epilepsy may already be on phenytoin. A lower loading dose should be given in these patients. Many of these patients will be having fits because of poor compliance. Oral **clomethiazole** or **chlordiazepoxide** is particularly useful where fits are due to alcohol withdrawal.

If the patient has not responded to prior therapy and seizure activity has lasted 1 h, the patient should be transferred to ICU and given a general anaesthetic (thiopentone or propofol) to abolish electrographic seizure activity and provide ventilatory support to prevent further cerebral damage. **Thiopentone** is a rapidly effective anticonvulsant in refractory status epilepticus and has cerebroprotective properties. Endotracheal intubation must be performed and the patient ventilated. Thiopentone has a number of pharmacokinetic disadvantages over propofol. Following an IV bolus, thiopentone is rapidly taken up in the brain, but high concentrations are not sustained due to its rapid redistribution into fatty tissues. For this reason an IV infusion should follow. Elimination of thiopentone may take days after prolonged infusion. Electroencephalographic monitoring is essential to ensure that the drug level is sufficient to maintain burst suppression. **Propofol**, although not licensed for the treatment of status epilepticus, has been used successfully. It certainly has pharmacokinetic advantages over thiopentone.

Paralysis with **suxamethonium**, **atracurium**, **vecuronium** or **pancuronium** is indicated if uncontrolled fitting causes difficulty in ventilation or results in severe lactic acidosis. Neuromuscular blockade should only be used in the presence of continuous EEG monitoring, as the clinical signs of seizure activity are abolished. Blind use of muscle relaxants without control of seizure activity may result in cerebral damage.

MANAGEMENT OF STATUS EPILEPTICUS

SHORT NOTES

TREATMENT OF STATUS EPILEPTICUS

Initial measures
- Position patient to avoid pulmonary aspiration of stomach contents
- Establish an airway (oropharyngenal or nasopharyngeal) and give 100% oxygen
- Monitor vital functions
- IV access
- Send bloods for FBC, U&E, calcium, glucose, anticonvulsant levels
- Arterial blood gas

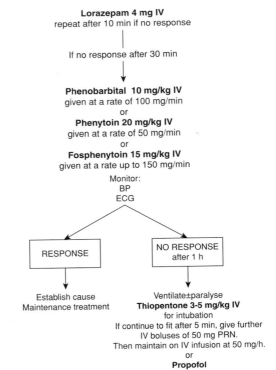

Lorazepam 4 mg IV
repeat after 10 min if no response

If no response after 30 min

Phenobarbital 10 mg/kg IV
given at a rate of 100 mg/min
or
Phenytoin 20 mg/kg IV
given at a rate of 50 mg/min
or
Fosphenytoin 15 mg/kg IV
given at a rate up to 150 mg/min

Monitor:
BP
ECG

RESPONSE

NO RESPONSE
after 1 h

Establish cause
Maintenance treatment

Ventilate±paralyse
Thiopentone 3-5 mg/kg IV
for intubation
If continue to fit after 5 min, give further
IV boluses of 50 mg PRN.
Then maintain on IV infusion at 50 mg/h.
or
Propofol

Monitor: EEG

Further investigations after stabilisation
- Serum magnesium
- LFTs
- CT±LP
- EEG

REASONS FOR TREATMENT FAILURE

There are several possible reasons for failure of treatment, most of which are avoidable:

- Inadequate emergency anticonvulsant therapy
- Failure to initiate maintenance anticonvulsant therapy
- Metabolic disturbance, hypoxia
- Cardiorespiratory failure, hypotension
- Failure to identify or treat underlying cause
- Other medical complications
- Misdiagnosis (pseudostatus)

PSEUDOSTATUS

Up to 30% of patients ventilated for 'status epilepticus' may have pseudo-status. Clinical features suggestive of pseudostatus are:

- More common in females
- History of psychological disturbance
- Retained consciousness during 'fits'
- Normal pupillary response to light during 'fits'
- Normal tendon reflexes and plantar responses immediately after 'fits'

The diagnosis may be aided by EEG monitoring and serum prolactin level – raised following a true fit. A normal prolactin level is not helpful in that it does not exclude status epilepticus.

PREVENTION OF DELIRIUM TREMENS AND ALCOHOL WITHDRAWAL SYNDROME

There are a variety of regimens available for this purpose. However, for many, **chlordiazepoxide** is the drug of choice. Sedative doses should be tailored to the individual requirements. This requires active titration at least once daily. Initial 30 mg four times daily should be adequate, but in severe cases, increase the dose to a maximum of 50 mg four times daily. For the night-time sedation, give a larger dose at bedtime for a quieter night!

Suggested oral regimen (titrate according to the patient's response):

	0800 hours	1200 hours	1800 hours	2200 hours
Day 1	30 mg	30 mg	30 mg	30 mg
Day 2	25 mg	25 mg	25 mg	25 mg
Day 3	20 mg	20 mg	20 mg	20 mg
Day 4	10 mg	10 mg	10 mg	20 mg
Day 5	5 mg	5 mg	5 mg	5 mg
Day 6	–	5 mg	5 mg	5 mg
Day 7	–	–	5 mg	5 mg
Day 8	–	–	–	5 mg

A smaller dose may be suitable (e.g. in the very elderly), in which case halve the doses. Prescribe 10–20 mg 'when required' in addition for breakthrough agitation.

Alternatives to chlordiazepoxide
- *Lorazepam* has a shorter duration of action than chlordiazepoxide and may be preferable in elderly patients or those with severe hepatic dysfunction (0.5 mg lorazepam ~15 mg chlordiazepoxide)
- *Diazepam* if the parenteral or rectal route is required (5 mg diazepam ~15 mg chlordiazepoxide)
- *Clomethiazole (chlormethiazole)* is useful if the patient is sensitive to benzodiazepines, but beware the increased risk of respiratory depression if the patient goes on an alcohol bender. A good regimen is to use Heminevrin® capsules (192 mg chlomethiazole): 3 capsules four times each day for day 1, 3 capsules three times daily for day 2, 2 capsules three times daily for day 3, 1 capsule four times daily for day 4, and 1 capsule three times daily for day 5. Do not discharge with any chlormethiazole.

Whatever drug and regimen is used, give a larger dose last thing at night, reduce doses if the patient is sleepy, and increase doses if signs of DTs are increasing.

Adjuncts to chlordiazepoxide

Continue any established antiepileptic drugs. For patients not on any anti-convulsants but known to be susceptible to seizures, prescribe carbamazepine 200 mg PO 12 hourly during detoxification. Use diazepam 10 mg IV/PR if chlordiazepoxide does not adequately control seizures. Consider propranolol 40 mg PO 8–12 hourly (or higher) when required for reducing sweating, palpitations and tremor if the patient is particularly distressed.

PREVENTION OF WERNICKE–KORSAKOFF SYNDROME

On admission, administer parenteral Pabrinex® (p. 176) to all alcohol-dependent patients undergoing inpatient alcohol withdrawal, or to those patients who are thought to be severely thiamine deficient. Pabrinex® contains vitamins B and C but we are using it for the thiamine content. Pabrinex® should be administered before any parenteral glucose is given.

Prevention of Wernicke's encephalopathy: ONE pair of Pabrinex® IVHP 5-ml ampoules once or twice daily for 3–5 days.

Therapeutic treatment for Wernicke's encephalopathy: TWO pairs of Pabrinex® IVHP ampoules three times daily for 3 days then review. If no response, discontinue therapy; if a response is seen, decrease dose to ONE pair daily given for as long as improvement continues.

When the Pabrinex® course is finished give oral thiamine 50 mg 8 hourly and multivitamins 1–2 tablets daily, usually for the rest of the admission. For severe vitamin B group deficiency, give vitamin B compound strong tablets 1–2 8 hourly. A short course of folic acid 5 mg PO daily may be beneficial.

ANTI-ARRHYTHMIC DRUGS

The traditional Vaughan Williams' classification (based on electrophysio-logical action) does not include anti-arrhythmic drugs such as digoxin and atropine. A more clinically useful classification categorises drugs according to the cardiac tissues which each affects, and may be of use when a choice is to be made to treat an arrhythmia arising from that part of the heart.

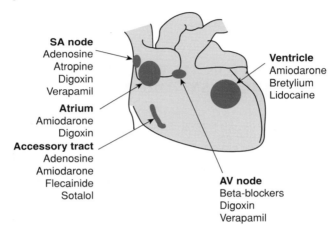

SA node
Adenosine
Atropine
Digoxin
Verapamil

Atrium
Amiodarone
Digoxin

Accessory tract
Adenosine
Amiodarone
Flecainide
Sotalol

Ventricle
Amiodarone
Bretylium
Lidocaine

AV node
Beta-blockers
Digoxin
Verapamil

INOTROPES AND VASOPRESSORS

Inotropes: receptors stimulated

Drug	Dose (µg/kg/min)	α_1	β_1	β_2	DA 1
Dopamine	1–5				+ +
	5–10		+	+	+ +
	>10	+	+	+	+ +
Dobutamine	1–25	0/+	+	+	
Dopexamine	0.5–6		0/+	+ + + +	+
Adrenaline	0.01–0.2	+/+ +	+	+	
Noradrenaline	0.01–0.2	+ + +	+		

Effects of inotropes

Drug	Cardiac contractility	Heart rate	SVR	Blood pressure	Renal and mesenteric blood flow
Dopamine:					
DA 1	0	0	0	0	+
β	+ +	+	0/+	+	0
α	0	0	+ +	+ +	−
Dobutamine	+ +	0	−	+	0
Dopexamine	0/+	+	−	0	+
Adrenaline	+ +	+	+/−	+	0/−
Noradrenaline	+	−	+ +	+ +	−

+, increase; 0, no change; −, decrease

Which inotrope to choose?

The definition of a positive inotrope is an agent that will increase myocardial contractility by increasing the velocity and force of myocardial fibre shortening.

All inotropes will, therefore, increase myocardial oxygen consumption. In the case of a normal coronary circulation, the increased oxygen demand caused by the increased inotropic state of the heart and the increase HR is met by increasing oxygen supply mediated by local mechanisms. In the presence of coronary artery disease, the increased oxygen demand may not be met by an increase in coronary blood flow. The tachycardia shortens the coronary diastolic filling time, reducing the coronary blood flow and making the ischaemia worse.

Therefore, inotropes have to be used with caution in patients with IHD.

The efficiency of the cardiac pump depends on preload, contractility, afterload and ventricular compliance. Each of these may be influenced by inotropes. In a patient with circulatory failure, an initial priority is to achieve an optimal preload by correcting any hypovolaemia. This may require the use of oesophageal Doppler monitoring or other minimally invasive monitoring techniques, which have largely superseded pulmonary artery catheterisation. If circulatory failure persists after optimal volume loading, a positive inotrope may be used to increase myocardial contractility. If intravascular volume has been restored (PCWP 10–15 mmHg) but perfusion is still inadequate, the selection should be based on the ability of the drug to correct or augment the haemodynamic deficit. If the problem is felt to be inadequate cardiac output, the drug chosen should have prominent activity at β_1 receptors and little activity. If the perfusion deficit is caused by a marked reduction in SVR, then a drug with prominent α activity should be used. The haemodynamic picture is often more complex than those presented above. Other special considerations such as oliguria, underlying ischaemic heart disease or arrhythmias may exist and affect the choice of drug.

Most inotropes increase contractility by increasing the intracellular Ca^{2+} concentration of cardiac cells. This may be achieved in three different ways.

- The catecholamines stimulate the β_1 receptor, which activates adenyl cyclase resulting in increased cAMP. This causes opening of Ca^{2+} channels.
- PDE inhibitors prevent the breakdown of cAMP, thus facilitating Ca^{2+} entry and uptake by the sarcoplasmic reticulum.
- Digoxin acts by inhibiting the Na^+/K^+ pump and increasing intracellular Ca^{2+} concentration indirectly through Na^+/Ca^{2+} exchange mechanism.

The other way to increase contractility is by increasing the sensitivity of the contractile protein troponin C to Ca^{2+}. Stretch and α-adrenergic stimulation increase the sensitivity of troponin C for Ca^{2+}.

Acidosis, hypoxia and ischaemia, on the other hand, decrease the sensitivity of troponin C for Ca^{2+} and, therefore, the force of contraction.

There is no one ideal inotrope. The choice of inotrope will be influenced by the cause of the circulatory failure. The catecholamines are the most frequently used inotropes in the ICU. All act directly on adrenergic receptors. There are currently considered to be two α-, two β- and five dopaminergic receptors. Adrenaline, noradrenaline and dopamine are naturally occurring catecholamines. Dopamine is the immediate precursor of noradrenaline, and noradrenaline is the precursor of adrenaline. Dobutamine is a synthetic analogue of isoprenaline that acts primarily on β-receptors in the heart. Dopexamine is a synthetic analogue of dopamine, acting primarily on β_2-receptors.

Adrenaline (epinephrine) has α and β activities. In low dose, β predominates and SVR may be reduced. With high doses, α-mediated vasoconstriction predominates.

There is no stimulation of dopamine receptors. Adrenaline is useful when there is a severe reduction in cardiac output (e.g. cardiac arrest), in which the arrhythmogenicity and marked increase in HR and myocardial oxygen consumption that occur with this drug are not limiting factors. It is the drug of choice in anaphylactic shock, due to its activity at β_1- and β_2-receptors and its stabilising effect on mast cells.

Noradrenaline (norepinephrine) is used to restore BP in cases of reduced SVR. The main haemodynamic effect of noradrenaline is predominantly α-mediated vasoconstriction. Noradrenaline can increase the inotropic state of the myocardium by α_1 and β_1 stimulation. The blood pressure is markedly increased due to vasoconstriction and the increase in myocardial contractility. However, cardiac output may increase or decrease due to the increase in afterload. The increase in blood pressure may cause reflex bradycardia. Noradrenaline will increase PVR. It is a potent vasoconstrictor of the renal artery bed. It also produces vasoconstriction in the liver and splanchnic beds with reduced blood flow. But in septic shock, noradrenaline may increase renal blood flow and enhance urine production by increasing perfusion pressure. It can be used to good effect in septic shock when combined with dobutamine to optimise oxygen delivery and consumption. It is essential that the patient is adequately filled before starting noradrenaline. Indiscriminate use of noradrenaline can aggravate the oxygen debt because of peripheral vasoconstriction.

Dopamine exerts its haemodynamic effects in a dose-dependent way. In low doses it increases renal and mesenteric blood flow by stimulating dopamine receptors. The increase in renal blood flow results in increased GFR and increased renal sodium excretion. Doses between 2.5 and 10 μg/kg/min stimulate β_1-receptors, resulting in increased myocardial contractility, stroke volume and cardiac output. Doses >10μg/kg/min stimulate α-receptors, causing increased SVR, decreased renal blood flow and increased potential for arrhythmias. The distinction between dopamine's predominant dopaminergic and α effects at low doses and β effects at higher doses is not helpful in clinical practice, due to marked interindividual variation. It may exert much of its effects by being converted to noradrenaline. However, because of overlap and individual variation, no dose is clearly only 'renal-dose' – dopaminergic effects may occur at higher doses, and vasoconstrictor effects at lower doses.

Dopamine tends to cause more tachycardia than dobutamine and unlike dobutamine usually increases rather than decreases pulmonary artery pressure and PCWP.

Dopamine has now been shown to have several adverse effects on other organ systems. On the respiratory system dopamine has been shown to reduce hypoxic respiratory drive and increase intrapulmonary shunt leading to decreased oxygenation. Dopamine depresses anterior pituitary function except for ACTH secretion. Prolactin, LH, GH and thyroid hormones are all suppressed. This will obtund the body's acute endocrine response to stress.

Dopamine may also alter immunological function via its inhibitory effect on prolactin secretion. Inhibition of prolactin causes humoral and cell-mediated immunosuppression.

With the current lack of evidence for renal protection and the numerous potential adverse effects, the use of low-dose dopamine for prevention of renal failure is no longer considered appropriate (Dellinger RP et al. *Int Care Med* 2013; **39**: 165–225).

Dobutamine has predominant β_1 activity. It is used when the reduced cardiac output is considered the cause of the perfusion deficit, and should not be used as the sole agent if the decrease in output is accompanied by a significant decrease in BP. This is because dobutamine causes reductions in preload and afterload, which further reduce the BP. If hypotension is a problem, noradrenaline may need to be added.

Dopexamine is the synthetic analogue of dopamine. It has potent β_2 activity with one-third the potency of dopamine on the DA_1 receptor, with little or no activity at α- and βl- adrenoceptors. Dopexamine increases HR and CO, causes peripheral vasodilatation, $\uparrow$ renal and splanchnic blood flow, and $\downarrow$ PCWP. The current interest in dopexamine is centred on its dopaminergic and anti-inflammatory activity. The anti-inflammatory activity and improved splanchnic blood flow may be due to dopexamine's β_2 rather than DA 1 effect. Recent studies including one carried out in the ICU in York have shown reduced mortality in patients undergoing major surgery in those pre-optimised to a protocol which included pre-operative fluid and inotrope administration to achieve a target oxygen delivery. Our study suggests that dopexamine is superior to adrenaline when used in the pre-optimised protocol. This may be attributable to improved organ perfusion and oxygen delivery to organs such as the gut and the kidneys. In comparison with other inotropes, dopexamine causes less increase in myocardial oxygen consumption.

This synthetic agonist has a number of different properties but is mainly a β_2-agonist. Dopexamine acts as a positive inotrope to increase the heart rate and decrease the systemic vascular resistance. In animals, dopexamine increases renal blood flow by DA_1 agonism to cause intrarenal vasodilatation, an increased cortical but not medullary blood flow and an increase in urine output. However, in man the effects on diuresis and natriuresis are small, and may solely reflect the increase in renal blood flow from the increased cardiac output. This results in an improved oxygen supply–demand balance compared with dopamine where the increased natriuresis is secondary to DA_2 activity, which increases oxygen requirements. Dopexamine also decreases gut permeability and may reduce bacterial translocation and endotoxinaemia.

There are two DA receptors with different functional activities (see table). Fenoldopam is a selective DA_1 agonist, introduced principally as an antihypertensive agent. It reduces blood pressure in a dose-dependent manner while preserving renal blood flow and GFR. As a DA_1 agonist, it acts postsynaptically to cause vasodilatation and so increase renal blood flow. Fenoldopam also improves creatinine clearance. It does not act as an inotrope, but is a selective vasodilator of both renal and mesenteric beds. Increasing doses of fenoldopam do not cause tachycardia or tachyarrhythmias, as the agent has no action on β- or α-receptors. However, a tachycardia may occur if there is rapid vasodilatation. It is not presently licensed in the UK. Use of fenoldopam was approved by the FDA for the treatment of accelerated hypertension in 1998; there has been increasing use of its renoprotective effects in doses ranging from 0.03 to 0.05 μg/kg/min.

Table: sites of action of dopaminergic receptor drugs and their agonist effects

Receptor	Site	Effects
DA_1	Renal and splanchnic beds	Vasodilatation, increased renal blood flow, natriuresis
DA_2	Postganglionic sympathetic nerves	Inhibits presynaptic norepinephrine release, decreases renal blood flow

Vasopressin

Vasopressin (antidiuretic hormone, ADH) controls water excretion in kidneys via V2 receptors and produces constriction of vascular smooth muscle via V1 receptors. In normal subjects vasopressin infusion has no effect on blood pressure but has been shown to significantly increase blood pressure in septic shock. The implication is that in septic shock there is a deficiency in endogenous vasopressin and this has been confirmed by direct measurement of endogenous vasopressin in patients with septic shock requiring vasopressors. In vitro studies show that catecholamines and vasopressin work synergistically. Anecdotally, use of 3 units/h is usually very effective and not associated with a reduction in urine output. As its pseudonym antidiuretic hormone implies, vasopressin infusion might be expected to decrease urine output but the opposite is the case at doses required in septic shock. This may be due to an increase in blood pressure and therefore perfusion pressure. It is also worth noting that, whereas noradrenaline constricts the afferent renal arteriole, vasopressin does not affect renal function. It has been shown that doses as high as 0.1 units/min (6 units/h) do reduce renal blood flow, so should be avoided. A dose of 0.04 units/ min (2.4 units/h) is often efficacious in septic shock and does not reduce renal blood flow. Vasopressin does not cause vasoconstriction in the pulmonary or cerebral vessels, presumably due to an absence of vasopressin receptors. It does cause vasoconstriction in the splanchnic circulation, hence the use of vasopressin in bleeding oesophageal varices. The dose required in septic shock is much lower than that required for variceal bleeding. It has been shown that doses as high as 0.1 units/min (6 units/h) do reduce renal blood flow, so should be avoided. A dose of 0.04 units/min (2.4 units/h) is often efficacious and does not reduce renal blood flow. Anecdotally, use of 3 units/h is usually very effective and not associated with a reduction in urine output. In septic shock, its use is reserved for cases where the requirement for noradrenaline exceeds 0.3 μg/kg/min. Vasopressin works synergistically with noradrenaline and as the patient's condition improves, the dose of vasopressin should be weaned down and off before the noradrenaline is stopped.

Enoximone and **milrinone** are both potent inodilators, and because they do not act via adrenergic receptors, they may be effective when catecholamines have failed. The inhibition of PDE III isoenzyme is responsible for the therapeutic effects. They can increase CO by 30–70% in patients with heart failure. They may also show synergy with catecholamines and have the added advantage of causing less ↑ myocardial oxygen consumption. Because they ↓ SVR and PVR, myocardial oxygen consumption is little increased compared with catecholamines. In addition they tend not to increase HR. There is also the added advantage of lusitropy – aiding relaxation of the ventricles and increasing coronary artery blood flow. The combination of inotropic support, vasodilatation, stable HR and improved diastolic relaxation is particularly advantageous in patients with IHD. Milrinone has an inotropy:vasodilatation ratio of 1:20 compared with 1:2 for enoximone. As a result, milrinone may need to be administered in combination with another inotrope or vasopressor.

The main use of enoximone and milrinone is the short-term treatment of severe congestive heart failure unresponsive to conventional therapy. In septic shock there is a significant risk of hypotension and they should be used with caution.

Digoxin has been used to treat heart failure for > 200 years. The inotropic effect of digoxin is largely due to increase in intracellular calcium produced indirectly by inhibition of the Na/K pump. Its role in acute heart failure is restricted to patients in fast AF. In the presence of high sympathetic activity, its inotropic effect is negligible. It has a low therapeutic index. The potential for toxicity in the critically ill patient is increased by hypokalaemia, hypomagnesaemia, hypercalcaemia, hypoxia and acidosis. Toxicity does not correlate with plasma levels and is manifested by all types of arrhythmias, including AF.

Levosimendan is a unique, currently unlicensed, agent which is used in some centres for patients with acute decompensated congestive heart failure (CHF). Levosimendan enhances myocardial contractility without increasing oxygen requirements, and causes coronary and systemic vasodilation. Studies have shown that levosimendan increases cardiac output and lowers cardiac filling pressures and is associated with a reduction of cardiac symptoms, risk of death and hospitalisation. Its action is independent of interactions with β-adrenergic receptors. Levosimendan's role in therapy remains unclear.

BRONCHOSPASM

Causes of wheezing in the ICU
- Pre-existing asthma/COPD
- Anaphylactic reaction
- Aspiration pneumonia
- Kinked tracheal tube
- Tracheal tube too far – carinal/bronchial stimulation
- Bronchial secretions
- Pulmonary oedema
- Pneumothorax

Signs of severe asthma needing intensive care
- Tachycardia (HR > 130/min)
- Pulsus paradox > 20 mmHg
- Tachypnoea (RR > 30/min)
- Absent wheezing
- Exhaustion
- Inability to complete a sentence
- $PaCO_2$ normal or increased
- Hypoxia

The selective β_2-agonists such as salbutamol and terbutaline are the treatment of choice for episodes of reversible bronchospasm. Patients with chronic bronchitis and emphysema are often described as having irreversible airways obstruction, but they usually respond partially to the β_2-agonists or to the antimuscarinic drugs ipratropium or oxitropium. There is some evidence that patients who use β_2-agonists on a 'PRN' basis show greater improvement in their asthma than those using them on a regular basis. In the critically ill these drugs will have to be given either nebulised or intravenously. The tracheobronchial route is preferable because the drug is delivered directly to the bronchioles; smaller doses are then required, which cause fewer side-effects. If the bronchospasm is so severe that very little drug gets to the site of action via the tracheobronchial route, then the drug will have to be given IV.

ANTI-ULCER DRUGS

Critically ill patients are highly stressed and this leads to an increased incidence of peptic ulceration. The risk of stress ulceration is increased in the presence of:

- Sepsis
- Head injury
- Major surgical procedures
- Multiple trauma
- Severe burn injuries
- Respiratory failure
- Severe hepatic failure
- Severe renal failure

Routine use of anti-ulcer drugs to all patients in an ICU is unnecessary. Use should be restricted to those who have the risk factors described above and should be stopped when patients are established on enteral feeding.

Patients who have a coagulopathy or on NSAIDs, SSRIs, clopidogrel or steroids (whether or not enterally fed) should be covered with a proton pump inhibitor (PPI) or ranitidine. The routine use of PPIs in the ICU is not justified; these are sometimes unintentionally continued long-term on discharge from ICU and are associated with *Clostridium difficile* infection.

IMMUNONUTRITION IN THE ICU

Patients admitted to the ICU may be malnourished at the time of admission, and certainly become so under the catabolic stress of major illness. The malnourished patient suffers from a reduction in immunity and is predisposed to infections. The importance of providing nutrition to critically ill patients is now widely accepted. Recently there has been a move to introduce certain dietary compounds with immune-enhancing actions to the feed. Compounds that have been found to have such properties include glutamine, arginine, nucleotides and omega-3 polyunsaturated fatty acids. None of these compounds when added into immune-enhancing enteral feeds have been shown to improve survival when compared with standard enteral feeds. However, most studies have shown reduction in infection rate, number of days ventilated and length of hospital stay. All these immune-enhancing formulas are significantly more expensive than standard formulas. In York, we supplement standard enteral feeds with glutamine (p. 110).

CORTICOSTEROIDS

While the normal physiological secretion of glucocorticoids from the adrenal cortex is about 30 mg cortisol per day, this can rise to 200–400 mg as part of the stress response to major surgery or trauma. Long-term therapy can suppress this adrenocortical response to stress. Patients on steroids or who have taken them within the past 12 months are also at risk of adrenal insufficiency. This may result in life-threatening hypotension, hyponatraemia and hyperkalaemia. The risk is greater when daily oral intake of prednisolone is >7.5 mg.

The aim in synthesizing new compounds has been to dissociate glucocorticoid and mineralocorticoid effects.

	Relative potencies		Equivalent dose (mg)
	Glucocorticoid	Mineralocorticoid	
Hydrocortisone	1	1	20
Prednisolone	4	0.25	5
Methylprednisolone	5	±	4
Dexamethasone	25	±	0.8
Fludrocortisone	10	300	–

In the critically ill patient, adrenocortical insufficiency should be considered when an inappropriate amount of inotropic support is required. Baseline cortisol levels and short synacthen test do not predict response to steroid. In patients who demonstrate a normal short synacthen test yet show a dramatic response to steroid, it is possible that the abnormality lies in altered receptor function or glucocorticoid resistance rather than abnormality of the adrenal axis. Baseline cortisol levels and short synacthen test are worthwhile to assess hypothalamic–pituitary–adrenal axis dysfunction versus steroid unresponsiveness.

However, the short synacthen test is no longer deemed necessary in septic shock management to identify those who might benefit from corticosteroid therapy. The use of steroid in septic shock remains controversial. The data suggests that hydrocortisone 50 mg IV 6 hourly is beneficial in resistant septic shock but not so in moderate septic shock. Higher doses of corticosteroids are associated with increased mortality in this indication.

SHORT SYNACTHEN TEST

Before starting corticosteroid treatment, it is worth confirming the diagnosis of adrenal insufficiency. Failure of plasma cortisol to rise after IM/IV tetracosactrin 250 μg indicates adrenocortical insufficiency.

Procedure:

- Contact lab first
- Take 5 ml blood in a plain tube for cortisol before and 30 min after IM/IV tetracosactrin 250 μg

Interpretation:

- A normal response requires an incremental rise of at least 200 nmol/l and a final result must be >500 nmol/l. In the critically ill, values should be much higher. We normally accept 1000 nmol/l anywhere in the test as being a level sufficient for a septic patient needing ventilatory support

The test is impossible to interpret once hydrocortisone has been started. If urgent treatment is required before test, use dexamethasone initially.

BONE MARROW RESCUE FOLLOWING NITROUS OXIDE

- Folic/folinic acid 15 mg IV for 2 days
- Vitamin B_{12} 1 mg IV for 2 days

The use of nitrous oxide for anaesthesia in excess of 2 h inactivates vitamin B_{12} and may lead to impaired DNA synthesis and megaloblastic bone marrow haemopoiesis. In fit patients this is of little significance, but in the critically ill it may increase the mortality rate. Haemopoeitic changes induced by nitrous oxide can be reversed by folic/folinic acid. Vitamin B_{12} is given to replace that which has been inactivated. It is recommended by some authorities that both folic/folinic acid and vitamin B_{12} should be given to critically ill patients following surgery in which nitrous oxide was used as part of the anaesthetic for >2 hours.

ANTIOXIDANTS

The human body in health constantly produces potentially harmful reactive oxygen species. These are balanced by complex antioxidant systems. Tissue injury is probably due, at least in part, to local imbalances in the oxidant/antioxidant ratio. This imbalance is called 'oxidative stress' and can cause lipid peroxidation, damage to DNA and cell death. Sources of oxidative stress during critical illness include reactive oxygen species produced by leucocytes ('respiratory burst') and production of nitric oxide by vascular endothelium. Studies have suggested that the total antioxidant potential of the plasma is decreased in septic patients who go on to develop organ dysfunction.

A logical, if simplistic, approach to the oxidative stress of critical illness has been the administration of agents with free radical scavenging properties. The hope is that the oxidant/antioxidant ratio will be restored towards normal and tissue damage will, therefore, be reduced. Agents that have been used for this purpose include acetylcysteine, vitamins A, C and E, zinc and selenium. There remains no confirmed benefit and the use of such agents must be viewed as speculative.

- Acetylcysteine (p. 4)
- Zinc (p. 241)
- Vitamin C (ascorbic acid)
  orally: 1 g daily dispersible tablets
  slow IV: 1 g daily (500 mg/5 ml)
- Vitamin E (tocopherol)
  orally: 100 mg 12 hourly (suspension 500 mg/5 ml)
  slow IV: 400 mg (oily injection 100 mg/2 ml)
- Selenium
  IV infusion: 400–800 µg sodium selenite daily in 50 ml sodium chloride 0.9%, given over 1–4 h. Normal range: 70–120 µg/l. 0.88–1.52 µmol/l.

POST-SPLENECTOMY PROPHYLAXIS

Following splenectomy, patients have a significantly increased risk of infection, predominantly by encapsulated organisms such as *Streptococcus pneumoniae*, *Haemophilus influenzae* and *Neisseria meningitidis*. Infection in patients with an absent or dysfunctional spleen remains largely preventable. Vaccinations and prophylactic antibiotics reduce but do not eliminate the risk of infection with these organisms. Patients should be educated about the potential risks of foreign travel, particularly with regard to malaria and unusual infections secondary to animal bites.

Vaccinations

Vaccine	Dose	Repeat dose
23-valent plain PPV (*Pneumovax II*)	0.5 ml by IM injection	Repeat every 5–10 years
Haemophilus influenzae type b (*Hiberix*)	0.5 ml by IM injection	No need
Meningitis C conjugate (*Meningitec* or *Menjugate*)	0.5 ml by IM or deep SC injection	No need
Annual influenza vaccine should be offered by the patient's GP.		

Where possible, the vaccines should be given 2 weeks before splenectomy. Otherwise, vaccination should optimally be given 2 weeks afterwards. This is because there is a dip in the immune response following major surgery. If it is not possible to organise this, a compromise is to vaccinate 3–5 days postoperatively (response suboptimal but adequate in most cases). It is preferable for each vaccine to be given into different limbs. Children less than 2 years of age respond poorly to the pneumococcal polysaccharide vaccine (PPV), so should receive pneumococcal conjugate vaccine (PCV).

Infection with serogroup C *N. meningitidis* accounts for around 40% of cases in the UK. No vaccine is currently available to protect patients against serogroup B *N. meningitidis*. The immunity conferred by the original meningococcal polysaccharide vaccine (*Mengivac A+C*) is not complete and is short-lived. Protection wanes rapidly and is generally gone by around 2 years from vaccination. The newer Meningitis C conjugate vaccines are more effective than polysaccharide vaccines and will provide long-term protection against infection. The Meningococcal ACWY conjugate vaccine (*Menveo*) is to be preferred over the Meningococcal ACWY polysaccharide vaccine (*ACWY Vax*).

Department of Health Green Book guidance, published December 2010, suggests differing vaccination regimens depending on patient age and prior vaccination status:

Patient age and vaccination status	DoH recommendation
Children <1 year of age	2 doses of MenACWY conjugate vaccine (*Menveo*) one month apart instead of the MenC vaccine in infancy FOLLOWED BY 1 dose of Hib/MenC vaccine at 12 months of age FOLLOWED BY 1 dose of MenACWY conjugate vaccine 2 months later
Children presenting when >1 year of age AND Adults	1 dose of Hib/MenC vaccine FOLLOWED BY 1 dose of MenACWY conjugate vaccine 2 months later
Children and adults who have been fully immunised with MenC vaccine as part of the routine programme	1 additional dose of the combined Hib/MenC vaccine FOLLOWED BY 1 dose of the MenACWY conjugate vaccine 2 months later

When travelling to a high-risk area for serogroup A, W135 or Y meningococcal disease, patients should receive the Meningococcal ACWY conjugate vaccine (*Menveo*).

Antibiotic prophylaxis
All patients should be given a stock of 'emergency' antibiotics. Lifelong prophylactic antibiotics should be offered to patients considered at continued 'high-risk' of pneumococcal infection. 'High-risk' patients are defined in current British Committee for Standards in Haematology (BCSH) guidelines as:

children <16 years old;
adults >50 years old;
splenectomy for haematological malignancy rather than trauma;
poor/no response to pneumococcal vaccine;
previous invasive pneumococcal infection.

Patients not at 'high-risk' should be counselled regarding the risks and benefits of lifelong antibiotics and may choose to discontinue them.

Oral penicillins remain the prophylactic drugs of choice in areas with low pneumococcal resistance. Specialist microbiological advice should be sought where this is not the case or for travel abroad. In patients with confirmed penicillin allergy, an appropriate macrolide may be substituted, depending on local practice.

Benzylpenicillin 600 mg 12 hourly IV

OR

Penicillin V 250 mg 12 hourly PO (omit if on cephalosporin prophylaxis for surgery)

OR

Erythromycin 500 mg 12 hourly IV or 250 mg 12 hourly PO (if confirmed penicillin allergy).

ANTI-MICROBIAL DRUGS

Use of anti-microbial agents causes predictable adverse effects, which have to be considered as part of a risk/benefit analysis for each individual patient, the intensive care unit as a whole and for the wider hospital environment. These effects include superinfection, selection of resistant microorganisms and toxic side-effects. Close liaison with a clinical microbiologist is important to ensure correct use of these agents in order to minimise these effects.

Anti-microbial agents may be used in the following ways:

- Prophylactic – to prevent an infective complication
- Empiric – to treat suspected infection before culture results are available
- Targeted – to treat established infection demonstrated by culture

Infection is only one of a number of causes of pyrexia in the intensive care unit setting (see below). Administration of anti-microbial agents to all febrile patients is not appropriate and will lead to significant overuse of these agents, often with multiple changes of anti-microbial in a futile attempt to get the temperature to settle. A daily ward round with a clinical microbiologist or infectious disease physician can help to avoid this problem and provide an opportunity to evaluate the significance of new microbiological culture results. It is particularly worth bearing in mind the phenomenon of drug fever which is commonly caused by antibiotics and results in a pyrexia which only resolves when the provoking agent is discontinued.

Non-infective causes of pyrexia

SIRS Trauma Burns Pancreatitis Acute hepatic failure
Thrombotic events such as DVT and PE
Myocardial infarction
Fibroproliferative phase of ARDS
Drugs
Antibiotics Hypnotics Diuretics Antihypertensives Antiarrhythmics NSAIDs Phenytoin

Blood/blood product transfusion
Cancer Lymphoma Leukaemia Hypernephroma Hepatoma Pancreatic carcinoma
Connective tissue disease Systemic lupus erythematosus Polyarteritis nodosa Polymyalgia/cranial arteritis
Sarcoidosis
Rheumatoid disease
Malignant hyperpyrexia

Empiric therapy should be reserved for those patients with well defined signs and symptoms of infection where delay in therapy would be expected to be harmful. It is essential to obtain appropriate specimens for microbiological examination, before starting empiric therapy. Requests for rapid tests, such as Gram stains and antigen detection techniques, and invasive sampling techniques, such as broncho-alveolar lavage (BAL) can be very helpful in guiding the need for empiric therapy and in modifying the choice of agents to be used.

The choice of agent(s) is also dependent on knowledge of the organisms likely to be involved. This should be based on previous experience within your own unit and should be designed to ensure coverage of the most likely pathogens, as failure to do so is associated with poorer patient outcomes. It should also take account of prior culture results for the individual patient concerned.

Anti-microbial therapy will not be successful in many infections associated with collections of pus or prosthetic devices without drainage or removal of the device as appropriate. Additional surgical intervention is not uncommonly required for intensive care unit patients.

Empiric therapy should be modified or stopped, as appropriate, once culture results become available. It is also good practice to have stop dates or review dates to avoid unnecessarily prolonged treatment or side-effects. Short course therapy of 5 to 7 days is adequate for most infections in the intensive care unit.

Although the majority of antibiotics are relatively safe drugs, important toxic effects do occur particularly in the presence of other disease states. In addition, antibiotics may result in secondary bacterial, yeast or fungal infection (superinfection), and may facilitate the growth of *Clostridium difficile*, a cause of diarrhoea and pseudomembranous colitis.

SHORT NOTES
ANTI-MICROBIAL DRUGS

Antibiotic resistance

Bacterial resistance to antibiotics is an established and increasing problem. Many pathogens are now 'multiresistant'. Excessive and inappropriate use of antibiotics is believed to be one of the most important factors in increasing the prevalence of antibiotic resistance. In most hospitals the intensive care unit has the highest prevalence of such organisms.

Staphylococcus aureus can survive for long periods in the environment and colonises the skin, nose or throat of approximately a third of patients and health care staff. If patients develop infections with *S. aureus*, this is usually by their own, commensal flora. *S. aureus* is readily spread either via hands or by contact with the inanimate environment. Methicillin-resistant *S. aureus* (MRSA), resistant to flucloxacillin, was first detected in Europe in the early 1960s.

Since 2008, data published by the European Antimicrobial Resistance Surveillance System (EARSS) has suggested a decreasing trend in the incidence of MRSA infections. This finding has been corroborated by the Health Protection Agency (HPA), which reports that counts and rates of MRSA bacteraemia continue to fall across the NHS. Between April 2011 and March 2012 (FY 2011/12), a total of 1,114 cases of MRSA bacteraemia were reported across the NHS. This equates to an MRSA bacteraemia rate of 2.1 per 100,000 bed-days and represents a 25% reduction on the 1,481 MRSA bacteraemia reports received in FY 2010/11. The introduction of routine screening for MRSA carriage was a significant turning point in the control of MRSA infection.

The majority of MRSA isolates in the UK belong to one of a relatively small number of epidemic strains, designated EMRSA-15 and EMRSA-16, which have spread widely throughout the country. In addition to inherent resistance to all beta-lactams (e.g. flucloxacillin), these strains usually express resistance to a number of antibiotics including macrolides and quinolones. Traditionally, glycopeptides (e.g. vancomycin and teicoplanin) have been used to treat infections with these organisms, although alternative antibiotics, including linezolid and daptomycin, are now available. Vancomycin-resistant *S. aureus* (VRSA) isolates have not yet been reported from cases in the UK but have emerged in other parts of the world. EARSS reports that, as of 2008, the only European country to have reported a case of VRSA is Austria. However, there is evidence that the minimal inhibitory concentration (MIC) of glycopeptide against *S. aureus* is rising. Given the MIC-dependent response of *S. aureus* to glycopeptides, this trend is of significant concern for the future.

MRSA is no longer the most important threat in terms of multi-drug resistance. Enterobacteriaceae such as *E. coli*, *Klebsiella* spp. and *Enterobacter* spp., expressing extended spectrum beta lactamases (ESBL) are being identified with increasing frequency, and have caused outbreaks in hospitals and the community. These organisms have markedly reduced susceptibilities to most commonly used penicillins and cephalosporins. As a result of growing problems with these organisms in the intensive care unit, empiric use of the carbapenems, including imipenem and meropenem, has increased. Unfortunately, resistance to the carbapenems is well established in *Pseudomonas aeruginosa* isolates, rising in *Acinetobacter* spp., and causing significant outbreaks in Enterobacteriaceae. There are few antibiotics left to treat significant infections with carbapenemase-producing Enterobacteriaceae, some of which are resistant to all β-lactams, fluoroquinolones, tigecycline, polymyxins and aminoglycosides. As such, the rise in antimicrobial resistance in Gram negative bacteria has recently led to significant media interest and has become a priority for the UK government. Quinolone-resistant strains of *Salmonella typhi* and *paratyphi* are being imported from the Indian sub-continent.

Penicillin-resistant *Streptococcus pneumoniae* are being isolated from cases of community-acquired pneumonia. In 2011, 0.8% of UK pneumococcal isolates tested resistant to penicillin, according to reports from the European Centre for Disease Prevention and Control (ECDC). Much higher rates of penicillin-resistant pneumococcal infections have been found in other European countries, particularly around the Mediterranean and in Eastern Europe. Five percent of UK isolates tested resistant to macrolides.

Enterococci form part of the normal human flora at multiple sites, particularly of the gastrointestinal tract, and can cause opportunistic infections. These organisms can grow and survive in harsh conditions and are inherently resistant to many classes of antibiotics, including cephalosporins and fluoroquinolones. *Enterococcus faecalis* is the most frequent species to be isolated, but *Enterococcus faecium* has the greater inherent resistance. Beta-lactams alone are ineffective against most strains of *E. faecium*.

EARSS reports that, over the last decades, enterococci have emerged as important nosocomial pathogens, paralleled by increases in glycopeptide and high-level aminoglycoside resistance. Vancomycin resistance in enterococci was first encountered in France and England but showed the most dramatic increase in the United States and was attributed to the widespread use of vancomycin. Since 2005, there has been a decreasing trend in glycopeptide resistance of enterococci in the UK. Conventional treatments of some serious enterococcal infections have involved the use of synergistic combinations of an aminoglycoside with a beta-lactam or a glycopeptide. *Enterococci* resistant to all synergistic combinations are now being reported.

Tuberculosis rates have been steadily rising in the UK. According to the HPA, there were 15.9 cases of tuberculosis per 100,000 population in the UK in 2011. Rates of multi-drug-resistant tuberculosis have been rising, accounting for 1.6% of new cases in 2011.

Clostridium difficile infection

Clostridium difficile is a Gram positive, spore-forming, toxin-producing, obligate anaerobic bacillus that is ubiquitous in nature. The spectrum of illness ranges from asymptomatic colonisation to diarrhoea (self-limiting to severe diarrhoea due to pseudomembranous colitis), toxic megacolon, colonic perforation and death. The increasing use of broad-spectrum antibiotics, sub-optimal infection prevention and control-related practices and the expanding population of patients with depressed immunity (including renal, oncology, haematology and intensive care patients) have resulted in an increase in the frequency of outbreaks of infection, which may be prolonged and difficult to control. *C. difficile* ribotype 0127 appears to be associated with poor outcome. *C. difficile* was first recognised as a significant cause of diarrhoea in the 1970s, with subsequent rates of disease rising markedly. Data published by the HPA shows that, since the introduction of mandatory *C. difficile* surveillance in the UK in 2007, disease rates have been declining.

Any antibiotic can cause *C. difficile* infection, including those used to treat the infection (i.e. vancomycin and metronidazole). Antibiotics particularly implicated include clindamycin, cephalosporins (particularly members of the third generation cephalosporins), quinolones (including ciprofloxacin) and co-amoxiclav. The most frequently implicated antibiotics causing *C. difficile* infection in the UK are amoxicillin and ampicillin, although this may also be a reflection of their high prescription rates. The standard treatment is oral/nasograstric metronidazole 400 mg 8 hourly or oral/nasogastric vancomycin 125 mg 6 hourly. Fidaxomicin is a newly licensed, expensive drug for this indication. It is a novel bactericidal macrocyclic antibiotic that inhibits bacterial ribonucleic acid polymerase. It is effective against *C. difficile* with limited activity against other Gram-positive bacteria. Two similar double-blind, randomised non-inferiority trials comparing oral vancomycin with fidaxomicin demonstrated no significant differences in clinical cure rates in the pre-specified subgroups of patients with severe or prior infection, but interestingly, recurrence rates were reduced with fidaxomicin. The high drug cost may be offset by the cost saved of treating additional episodes.

BACTERIAL GRAM STAINING

	Positive	Negative
COCCI	*Enterococcus* spp. *Staphylococcus* spp. *Streptococcus* spp. *Streptococcus pneumoniae*	*Moraxella catarrhalis* *Neisseria* spp.
RODS	*Actinomyces israelii* *Clostridium* spp. *Corynebacterium diphtheriae* *Listeria monocytogenes*	*Bacteroides* spp. *Burkholderia cepacia* *Enterobacter* spp. *Escherichia coli* *Haemophilus influenzae* *Klebsiella pneumoniae* *Legionella pneumophila* *Proteus mirabilis* *Pseudomonas aeruginosa* *Salmonella* spp. *Serratia marcescens* *Shigella* spp. *Stenotrophomonas*

ANTIBIOTICS: SENSITIVITIES

Column headers:

Staphylococcus aureus · MRSA · Streptococcus pyogenes · Streptococcus · Enterococcus faecalis · Enterococcus faecium · Haemophilus influenzae · Escherichia coli · ESBL positive E. coli · Klebsiella spp. · Neisseria meningitidis · Proteus spp. · Moraxella catarrhalis · Serratia spp. · Pseudomonas · Bacteroides fragilis · Clostridium perfringens · Clostridium difficile

Antibiotics (rows):

- Amoxicillin
- Ampicillin
- Benzylpenicillin
- Cefuroxime
- Cefotaxime
- Ceftazidime
- Ceftriaxone
- Ciprofloxacillin
- Clarithromycin
- Clindamycin
- Co–amoxiclav
- Erythromycin
- Flucloxacillin
- Gentamicin
- Imipenem
- Levofloxacin
- Linezolid
- Meropenem
- Metronidazole
- Tazocin
- Teicoplanin
- Timentin
- Trimetoprim
- Vancomycin

Legend:

- ■ Usually sensitive
- ▨ *Many strains resistant*
- ☐ Resistant or not recommended

When referring to this chart it is important to bear in mind the following:

- Antibiotic susceptibility is reducing in many organisms. There are great geographical variations in antibiotic resistance, not only between different countries, but also between different hospitals
- There may be a significant difference between antibiotic susceptibility determined in vitro and the clinical response, in vivo
- Gram-positive bacteria are intrinsically resistant to aztreonam, temocillin, polymyxin B/colistin and nalidixic acid
- Flucloxacillin may have activity against *S. pneumoniae* but it is not used to treat pneumococcal pneumonia
- Most staphylococci are penicillinase producers
- Methicillin-resistant *S. aureus* (MRSA) isolates are resistant to beta-lactam agents, including beta lactamase inhibitor combinations, except for cephalosporins with approved anti-MRSA activity and clinical breakpoints (e.g. ceftaroline and ceftobiprole)
- Enterobacteriaceae are intrinsically resistant to benzylpenicillin, glycopeptides, fusidic acid, lincosamides, streptogramins, rifampicin, daptomycin and linezolid. They are also resistant to macrolides, although azithromycin is effective in vivo for the treatment of typhoid fever and erythromycin may be used to treat travellers' diarrhoea
- Extended spectrum beta-lactamase (ESBL) producers are often categorised as susceptible to combinations of a penicillin and a beta-lactamase inhibitor. With the exception of urinary tract infections and bloodstream infections secondary to this origin, the use of these combinations in infections caused by ESBL producers remains controversial and should be approached with caution
- Non-fermentative gram-negative bacteria are intrinsically resistant to benzylpenicillin, cefoxitin, cefamandole, cefuroxime, glycopeptides, fusidic acid, macrolides, lincosamides, streptogramins, rifampicin, daptomycin and linezolid
- *Burkholderia cepacia* and *Stenotrophomonas maltophilia* are intrinsically resistant to all aminoglycosides
- *Stenotrophomonas maltophilia* is typically susceptible to trimethoprim–sulphamethoxazole but resistant to trimethoprim alone
- *N. meningitidis* is susceptible to imipenem but it would not be used for treatment because of neurotoxicity (risk of convulsions)
- Although ciprofloxacin is not used for treatment of meningitis, HPA guidance for public health management of meningococcal disease in the UK recommends its use as prophylaxis for contacts (not licensed)

RENAL REPLACEMENT THERAPY

Techniques available

Renal support in intensive care varies substantially between units. In the early days of intensive care, renal support was limited to either **haemo-dialysis** or **peritoneal dialysis**. Advances in membrane technology led to the development of 'continuous arteriovenous haemofiltration' (CAVH). The driving pressure in this system is the patient's blood pressure; the blood is taken from an artery and returned to a vein. An ultrafiltrate of plasma water is produced, which is replaced by 'replacement fluid' that resembles plasma water but is devoid of the 'unwanted' molecules and ions, such as urea, creatinine and potassium. Fluid removal is achieved by replacing only a proportion of the volume of the fluid filtered. The development of CAVH enabled renal support to be undertaken on intensive care even in the absence of facilities for haemodialysis.

CAVH is now rarely used because of its problems, which include the dependence on systemic blood pressure, the need for large-bore arterial access and, even when running optimally, poor clearances. Some of these problems have been at least partly overcome by the development of the now most commonly used renal replacement technique used in the critically ill; 'continuous veno-venous haemofiltration' (CVVH).

Peritoneal dialysis has limited use in critically ill patients. It is efficient at fluid removal but is inefficient at removal of toxic solutes and is often completely inadequate in the catabolic critically ill patient. Protein loss, hyperglycaemia, risk of infection and diaphragmatic splinting further contribute to its limited use in the critically ill.

In continuous veno-venous haemofiltration (**CVVH**), blood is removed and returned into large-bore venous access by use of a mechanical pumping system. The higher blood flow rates achievable mean greater clearances, even in the presence of systemic hypotension, and the use of double-lumen central venous catheters has reduced the problems of vascular access. The simplicity of CAVH has been lost as the use of a mechanical pump has made necessary pressure monitors for the limbs of the vascular access, a bubble trap and an air detector. Incorporated in modern systems are also systems for measuring the filtrate, adjusting and infusing the replacement fluid and infusing anti-coagulants. A further refinement is the use of **haemodiafiltration**, in which an element of dialysis is added to the clearance of solute by haemofiltration. In haemofiltration the membrane acts like a sieve in which plasma water is lost through the membrane pores, driven by the transmembrane pressure gradient. The membrane allows passage of molecules up to about 30 000 daltons molecular weight, although other factors such as charge and plasma protein binding will also affect clearance. In dialysis a dialysate is passed in the opposite direction to the flow of blood. The membrane used for dialysis is of smaller pore size than that used for haemofiltration and allows clearance of molecules up to about 500 daltons. In haemodiafiltration, a haemofiltration membrane is used and a dialysate fluid (often more haemofiltration replacement fluid) is pumped countercurrent to the blood flow through the filtrate space. The filtrate and dialysate fluid are collected together. The use of the dialysate particularly increases the clearance of the lower molecular weight molecules, such as urea (60 daltons) and creatinine (113 daltons).

Early reports of haemodialysis described marked haemodynamic instability in critically ill patients with its use and this contributed to the predominance of haemofiltration in the renal support of the critically ill. More recent reports demonstrate a reduction in haemodynamic instability with the use of modern membranes and techniques. The exact technique used for renal support in the critically ill depends on local policy and availability.

There is continuing interest in the ability of haemofiltration to remove so-called 'middle molecules'. These are molecules that are too large to be cleared by conventional haemodialysis, but are demonstrably cleared by haemofiltration. These include molecules such as TNF α (molecular weight 16 500 daltons). Whether the removal of these molecules with high flow haemofiltration reaches clinically significant levels of clearance and leads to clinical benefit remains controversial.

Haemofiltration membranes are made of synthetic polymers such as polysulfone or polyacrylonitrile. These are supplied as a cylindrical canister in which there are several thousand hollow fibres held within a plastic casing. The blood passes down the middle of the hollow fibres with filtrate emerging into the space between the fibres.

Composition of haemofiltration replacement fluid:

Sodium	140 mmol/l
Chloride	115 mmol/l
Calcium	1.75 mmol/l
Magnesium	0.75 mmol/l
Sodium lactate	3.36 g/l
Dextrose	1 g/l
Potassium	nil (may need to be added)
Phosphate	nil
Osmolarity	293 mosm/l

Composition of lactate-free replacement fluid:

Sodium	110 mmol/l
Chloride	115 mmol/l
Calcium	1.75 mmol/l
Magnesium	0.75 mmol/l

In exceptional circumstances, lactate-free haemodiafiltration with systemic IV infusion of sodium bicarbonate may be needed in severe liver disease or lactic acidosis. Failure to infuse sodium bicarbonate will result in severe hyponatraemia and worsening acidosis, as the patient's own bicarbonate is filtered out. The sodium bicarbonate requirement is

30 mmol per litre of replacement fluid or 750 mmol per 25-litre exchange. Remember that 1 ml of 8.4% sodium bicarbonate solution is equivalent to 1 mmol sodium and 1 mmol bicarbonate.

Creatinine clearances and dose calculation

The clearances achieved by renal replacement therapies are very variable, but roughly are in the region of:

Technique	Creatinine clearance (ml/min)
CAVH	9
CVVH	See text below
CVVHD	
IHD	160
PD	3

CVVHD = continuous veno-venous haemodiafiltration
IHD = intermittent haemodialysis
PD = peritoneal dialysis

The much higher clearances with haemodialysis allow intermittent treatment. Some units use a large haemofilter with high flow rates and achieve much higher clearances, which allows intermittent haemofiltration. Adequate clearances can be achieved with lower performance techniques if used continuously.

For haemofiltration, the clearance achieved is variable and is dependent on the ultrafiltration rate, the blood flow rate, the amount of pre-dilution and the haemocrit count.

$$\text{Clearance} = (\text{Sieving coef.}) \times (\text{total ultrafiltration rate}) / (1 + (\text{Predilution flow rate})/(\text{plasma flow rate}))$$

where plasma flow = blood flow × (1–haematocrit)

For example (1) A haemofiltered patient with the following settings, post-dilution of 700 ml/h, pre-dilution of 200 ml/h, blood flow of 200 ml/min and Hct of 0.25. Assuming sieving coefficient of 1. Plasma flow rate = 150 ml/min (blood flow 200 ml/min and Hct 0.25).

Total haemofiltration rate of 1000 ml/60 mins = 17 ml/min

Pre-dilution flow rate = 300 ml/60 mins = 5 ml/min
Clearance = 17/(1 + 5/150) = 16.5 ml/min.

Therefore, these settings provide a clearance of 16.5 ml/min.

Example (2) A haemofiltered patient with the following settings, pre-dilution 1 l/h, post-dilution 500 ml/h, blood flow 220 ml/min with a haemocrit of 0.26. Assuming sieving coefficient of 1, 150 ml/min (blood flow 220 ml/min and Hct 0.26), provides a clearance of approximately 22 ml/min

$$25/(1 + 21/163) = 22.1 \text{ ml/min.}$$

A pragmatic approach to dosing in haemofiltration is to calculate the clearance produced by the filter as described earlier, and then to dose the drug in relation to this clearance. The advantage of this approach is that it allows for the variety of filtration rates that are used in practice. This approach provides a patient-specific optimised approach rather than the more traditional fixed dosing tables.

For example

An 80 kg patient is being haemofiltered with the following settings, pre-dilution 1 l/h, post-dilution 500 ml/h, blood flow 220 ml/min with a haemocrit of 0.26.

The patient needs to be treated for herpes simplex encephalitis with aciclovir.

Consulting the aciclovir monograph in this book, we note that the dose for CC 10–25 is 5–10 mg/kg every 24 hours depending on indication (i.e. 5 mg/kg for HSV, HZV; 10 mg/kg for HZV in immuno-compromised, HSE). Therefore, we prescribe aciclovir 800 mg (10 mg/kg) once daily.

However, two days later the filter rate is increased to 2 l/h post-dilution and 500 ml pre-dilution and the pump speed increased to 250 ml/min, while the Hct is unchanged. The new rate of clearance calculated, using the method described here, is 40 ml/min and, consequently, the dose is increased to 800 mg every 12 hours (as the monograph suggests the frequency is 12 hourly if the CC is between 20–50 ml/min).

However, do not be a slave to the dosing calculations described here. It is not an exact science. There is a place for using clinical judgement to perhaps increase the dose for obese patients and aggressive anti-infective treatment in the first few days of treatment. Additionally, breaks in continuous therapy will have an impact on drug clearance.

EXTRACORPOREAL DRUG CLEARANCE: BASIC PRINCIPLES

- Extracorporeal elimination is only likely to be significant if its contribution to total body clearance exceeds 25–30%
- Neither renal failure nor renal replacement therapy requires adjustment of the loading dose. This depends on the volume of distribution
- The maintenance doses of drugs that are normally substantially cleared by the kidneys should be adapted to the effective clearance of the replacement therapy of the particular drug
- Extracorporeal elimination only replaces glomerular filtration (i.e. no tubular secretion or reabsorption). As a consequence there are potential inaccuracies in using the creatinine clearance of a replacement therapy as a basis of drug dosage calculation
- If the volume of distribution is large, changes in tissue concentration due to extracorporeal elimination will be small
- Only free drug in plasma can be removed
- Other factors affecting clearance include:
  - the molecular weight of the drug
  - the lipid solubility of the drug
  - the permeability and binding characteristics of the membrane
  - the actual technique employed (such as dialysis or filtration)
- For haemofiltration it is customary to refer to the 'sieving coefficient'.

$$\text{Sieving coefficient (S)} = \frac{\text{concentration in ultrafiltrate}}{\text{concentration in plasma}}$$

For urea and creatinine the sieving coefficient = 1 Elimination of drugs by any extracorporeal system will vary according to the details of the technique used, such as the membrane surface area, blood flow rate, duration of cycle.

The clearance of any drug by pure haemofiltration (clearance by 'convection' Cl_{HDF}) is, therefore, obtained by multiplying the sieving coefficient by the ultrafiltration rate (Q_F volume of filtration per unit time):

$$Cl_{HDF} = S \times Q_F$$

DRUG DOSES IN RENAL FAILURE/ RENAL REPLACEMENT THERAPY

It is convenient to divide drugs into four groups:

- Those requiring no dose reduction in renal failure
- Those that may require a dose reduction in renal failure
- Those requiring no further dose modification during renal replacement therapy
- Those that may require further dose modification due to renal replacement therapy

Drugs requiring NO DOSE MODIFICATION in renal failure

Acetylcysteine	Heparin
Adenosine	Hydrocortisone
Adrenaline	Insulin
Alfentanil	Ipratropium
Amiodarone	Isoprenaline
Amitryptiline	Labetolol
Atracurium	Lactulose
Atropine	Lignocaine
Calcium	Loperamide
Ceftriaxone	Methylprednisolone
Chlormethiazole	Naloxone
Ciclosporin	Nifedpine
Cyclizine	Nimodipine
Desmopressin	Noradrenaline
Dexamethasone	Nystatin
Dobutamine	Ondansetron
Dopamine	Phentolamine
Dopexamine	Phenytoin
Doxapram	Propofol
Epoetin	Protamine
Epoprostenol	Salbutamol
Esmolol	Suxamethonium
Fentanyl	Thiopentone
Flumazenil	Vecuronium
Glutamine	Verapamil
Glycerol suppository	Vitamin K
Granisetron	Zinc

DOSE MODIFICATION for haemofiltration therapy and renal failure

CC (ml/min)	<10	10–25	25–50	Dose in normal renal function
Aciclovir (IV)[1]	2.5–5 mg/kg every 24 hours depending on indication (i.e. 2.5 mg/kg for HSV, HZV; 5 mg/kg for HZV in immunocompromised, HSE)	5–10 mg/kg every 24 hours depending on indication (i.e. 5 mg/kg for HSV, HZV; 10 mg/kg for HZV in immunocompromised, HSE)	5–10 mg/kg every 12 hours depending on indication (i.e. 5 mg/kg for HSV, HZV; 10 mg/kg for HZV in immunocompromised, HSE)	5–10 mg/kg every 8 hours depending on indication (i.e. 5 mg/kg for HSV, HZV; 10 mg/kg for HZV in immunocompromised, HSE)

CC (ml/min)	<10	10–20	20–50	
Amikacin[1]	2 mg/kg every 24–48 hours	3–4 mg/kg every 24 hours	5–6 mg/kg every 12 hours	7.5 mg/kg every 12 hours or
	Measure peak and trough levels. Do NOT withhold next dose awaiting results from lab. as this risks underdosing			15 mg/kg every 24 hours; then adjusted according to levels
Aminophylline[1]	IV and oral: 100% of normal dose and adjust in accordance with blood levels			Modified release: 225–450 mg every 12 hours IV loading dose: 5 mg/kg (250–500 mg) Maintenance dose: typically 0.5 mg/kg/hour adjusted according to levels

CC (ml/min)	<10	10-20	20-50	Dose in normal renal function
Ambisome (Amphotericin liposomal)[1]		100% of normal dose		1-3 mg/kg/day maximum 5 mg/kg (unlicensed dose)
Benzylpenicillin[1]	600 mg-1.2 g every 6 hours*	600 mg-2.4 g every 6 hours*	100% of normal dose	2.4-14.4 g daily in 4-6 divided doses
Caspofungin[1]		100% of normal dose		70 mg loading dose on day 1 followed by 50 mg daily, thereafter If patient weighs >80 kg use 70 mg daily, severe liver failure use 35 mg daily.

CC (ml/min)	6-15	16-30	31-50	
Ceftazidime[1]	1 g every 24 hours (every 48 hours if CC<5 ml/min)	1 g every 12 hours	2 g every 12 hours	2 g every 8 hours

CC (ml/min)	<10	10-20	20-50	
Ceftriaxone[1]	2 g every 24 hours	2 g every 12 hours	2 g every 12 hours	Severe infections: 2-4 g every 24 hours
Cefuroxime (IV)[1]	750 mg-1.5 g every 12-24 hours*	750 mg-1.5 g every 8-12 hours*	750 mg-1.5 g every 8 hours*	Parenteral: 750 mg-1.5 g every 6-8 hours

(Continued)

307

CC (ml/min)	<19	20–29	30–40	41–55	
Cidofovir[3]	0.5 mg/kg weekly	1 mg/kg weekly 1.5 mg/kg weekly	1 mg/kg weekly	2 mg/kg weekly	
CC (ml/min)	<10	10–20	10–20	20–50	
Ciprofloxacin[1]	50% of normal dose (100% dose may be given for short periods under exceptional circumstances)	100% of normal dose			Oral: 250–750 mg every 12 hours IV: 100–400 mg every 12 hours
CC (ml/min)	<10	10–30	10–30	30–50	
Clarithromycin (IV and Oral)[1]	100% of normal dose				Oral: 250–500 mg every 12 hours IV: 500 mg every 12 hours
CC (ml/min)	<10	10–20	10–20	20–50	
Clindamycin[1]	100% of normal dose				*Dose in normal renal function* Oral: 150–450 mg every 6 hours, Endocarditis prophylaxis: 600 mg 1 hour before procedure IV: 0.6–4.8 g every 24 hours in 2–4 divided doses, Prophylaxis: 300 mg 15 minutes before procedure then 150 mg 6 hours later

CC (ml/min)	<10	10-30	30	
Co-amoxiclav[1][2]	IV: initial dose of 1.2 g and then 600 mg every 24 hours[2] Oral: 100% of normal dose[1]	IV: initial dose of 1.2 g and then 600 mg every 12 hours[2] Oral: 100% of normal dose[1]	IV and oral: 100% of normal dose	IV: 1.2 g every 8 hours Oral: 625 mg (one tablet) every 8 hours

CC (ml/min)	<10	10-20	20-50	
Colistin[1]	IV: 1 million units every 18-24 hours	IV: 1 million units every 12-18 hours or 50% of dose	IV: 2 million units every 8 hours	IV: <60 kg: 0.05-0.075 million units/kg split into 3 divided doses every 8 hours >60 kg 1-2 million units every 8 hours Nebulised solution: 1-2 million units every 12 hours

Neb[3]: decreased dose; use with caution (serum concentration estimations are recommended)

CC (ml/min)	<15	15-30	30-50	
Co-trimoxazole (80 mg trimethoprim/400 mg sulfamethoxazole)[1][4]	Haemodialysis required 50% of normal dose for both PCP and non-PCP treatment	PCP: normal dose for 3 days, then reduce by 50% for remainder of treatment course[4] Non-PCP: 50% of normal dose[1]	100% of normal dose	*Dose in normal renal function* PCP: 120 mg/kg/day for 2 days then reduced to 90 mg/kg/day for a further 19 days, given in 2-4 divided doses[2] Oral PCP prophylaxis: 480-960 mg daily or 960 mg on alternate days or twice daily Mondays, Wednesday and Fridays. Acute exacerbations of chronic bronchitis and urinary tract infections on microbiological advice: IV: 960 mg-1.44 g every 12 hours Oral: 960 mg every 12 hours[1]

(Continued)

CC (ml/min)	<10	10–20	20–50	
Digoxin[1]	62.5 µg alternate days or 62.5 µg daily, monitor levels	125–250 µg per day monitor levels	125–250 µg per day monitor levels	
Erythromycin[1]	50%–75% of normal dose, max. 2 g daily	100% of normal dose		Prokinetic: IV: 250–500 mg every 6 hours Oral: 250–500 mg every 6 hours
Flucloxacillin[1]	100% of normal dose up to a total daily dose of 4 g	100% of normal dose		Oral: 250–500 mg every 6 hours IV: 250 mg–2 g every 6 hours Endocarditis: max. 2 g every 4 hours if >85 kg Osteomyelitis: max. 8 g daily in divided doses

CC (ml/min)	<10	10–20	20–50	
Fluconazole[1]	50% of normal dose	100% of normal dose; if haemofiltered: increase treatment dose to 800 mg every 24 hours[6]		Dose in normal renal function 50–400 mg every 24 hours
Foscarnet sodium		see local guidelines		
Fusidic acid/sodium fusidate (IV/NG/PO)[1]		100% of normal dose		Oral: 500 mg (as sodium fusidate) every 8 hours Suspension: 750 mg every 8 hours (as fusidic acid) IV: 500 mg (as sodium fusidate) every 8 hours

CC (ml/min)	<10	10–25	26–50	
Ganciclovir[3]	1.25 mg/kg x 3 per week (or after haemodialysis)	1.25 mg/kg/day	2.5 mg/kg/day	CMV infection: Treatment (IV infusion): Induction: 5 mg/kg every 12 hours for 14–21 days
CC (ml/min)	5–10	10–20	21–70	
Gentamicin	2 mg/kg every 48–72 hours according to levels[1]	Loading dose 2 mg/kg then 80 mg every 12 hours[5]	7 mg/kg every 24 hours or 80 mg every 8 hours[5]	
		and monitor levels		
CC (ml/min)	<10	10–20	20–50	
Itraconazole	Oral: 100% of normal dose[1] Although oral bioavailability may be lower in renal insufficiency[2] IV: 100% of normal dose[1] Hydroxypropyl-β-cyclodextrin is a component of the IV preparation, which is eliminated through glomerular filtration. If CC is <30 ml/min, the IV formulation is contraindicated[2]; although in practice this is frequently ignored without apparent problems			100–200 mg every 12–24 hours according to indication
Linezolid[1]	100% of normal dose (monitor closely if CC<10 ml/min)			600 mg every 12 hours

(Continued)

CC (ml/min)	<10	10–20	20–50	Dose in normal renal function
Meropenem[1]	500 mg–1 g every 24 hours*	500 mg–1 g every 12 hours* or 500 mg every 8 hours*	500 mg–2 g every 12 hours*	500 mg–1 g every 8 hours. 500 mg is the standard dose; 1 g is used for resistant *Klebsiella* & ESBL. Higher doses used in cystic fibrosis and meningitis (up to 2 g every 8 hours)
Metronidazole[1]		100% of normal dose		Oral: 200–400 mg every 8 hours IV: 500 mg every 8 hours PR: 1 g every 8–12 hours
Midazolam	Use minimum dose and titrate to sedation score			
Morphine[1]	Use small doses, e.g. 1.25–2.5 mg and extended dosing intervals. Titrate according to response	Use small doses, e.g. 2.5–5 mg and extended dosing intervals. Titrate according to response	75% of normal dose	5–20 mg every 4 hours (higher in very severe pain or terminal illness)

CC (ml/min)	<10	10–30	30	
Oseltamivir[7]	Treatment: 75 mg STAT repeated every 5 days if required. Prophylaxis: 30 mg STAT every 7 days (usually 2 doses)	Treatment: 75 mg once to twice daily Prophylaxis: 75 mg every second day	Treatment:75–150 mg 12 hourly Prophylaxis: 75 mg once daily	Treatment 75–150 mg PO 12 hourly: usually for 5 days, can be extended Prophylaxis: usually for 10 days

CC (ml/min)	<10	10-20	20-50	Dose in normal renal function
Piperacillin/ Tazobactam (Tazocin)[1]	4.5 g every 12 hours	4.5 g every 8 hours	4.5 g every 8 hours	2.25-4.5 g every 6-8 hours
CC (ml/min)	<10	10-20	20-50	
Posaconazole[1]		100% of normal dose		400 mg every 12 hours with food or 240 ml of a nutritional supplement or 200 mg every 6 hours without food Oropharyngeal candidiasis severe infection or in immunocompromised patients: Loading dose of 200 mg (5 ml) once on the first day then 100 mg (2.5 ml) every 24 hours for 13 days Prophylaxis of invasive fungal infections: 200 mg every 8 hours

(Continued)

	<10	10-20	20-50	Dose in normal renal function
Propofol[1]	100% of normal dose			Sedation: 0.3-4 mg/kg/h
Ranitidine[1]	50%-100% of normal dose	100% of normal dose		Oral: 150-300 mg every 12-24 hours Zollinger Ellison: 150 or 300 mg every 8 hours IV injection: 50 mg every 6-8 hours
Teicoplanin[1]	Give normal loading dose, then 200-400 mg every 48-72 hours	Give normal loading dose, then 400 mg every 48 hours	Give normal loading dose, then 100% of maintenance dose	Loading dose: 400 mg every 12 hours for 3 doses, then IV: 400 mg daily, or 3-6 mg/kg/day (up to 10 mg/kg/day in some reports) in life-threatening infections
Tranexamic acid[1]	IV: 5 mg/kg every 12-24 hours Oral: 12.5 mg/kg every 12-24 hours	IV: 10 mg/kg every 12-24 hours Oral/ng: 25 mg/kg every 12-24 hours	IV: 10 mg/kg every 12 hours Oral: 25 mg/kg every 12 hours	

CC (ml/min)	<20	20–29	30–39	40–54	55–74	75–89	90–110	Dose in normal renal function
Vancomycin[8]	IV: 500 mg every 48 hours	IV: 500 mg every 24 hours	IV: 750 mg every 24 hours	IV: 500 mg every 12 hours	IV: 750 mg every 12 hours	IV: 1 g every 12 hours	IV: 1.25 g every 12 hours	IV: LD (independent of renal function) based on actual body weight: <60 kg 1 g, 60–90 kg 1.5 g, >90 kg 2 g, then maintenance dose: if CrCL >110 1.5 g 12 hourly, if Cr <111 then according to table.
	Oral: 100% of normal dose	Oral/ng: 100% of normal dose	Oral/ng: 100% of normal dose	Oral/ng: 100% of normal dose	Oral/ng: 100% of normal dose	Oral/ng: 100% of normal dose	Oral: 100% of normal dose	Oral: 125 mg or 500 mg every 6 hours (higher dose for resistant cases of *Clostridium difficile*)

(Continued)

. CC (ml/min)	<15	15–30	30–50	50–79	Dose in normal renal function
Voriconazole[1]			100% of normal dose		IV: 6 mg/kg every 12 hours for 24 hours, then 3–4 mg/kg every 12 hours Oral:<40 kg, 200 mg (5 ml) every 12 hours for 24 hours, then 100–150 mg every 12 hours >40 kg, 400 mg (10 ml) every 12 hours for 24 hours, then 200–300 mg every 12 hours
Zanamivir (IV)[7] Unlicensed product	Initial dose: 600 mg and 48 hours later, maintenance dose: 60 mg BD	Initial dose: 600 mg and 24 hours later, maintenance dose: 150 mg BD	Initial dose: 600 mg and 12 hours later, maintenance dose: 250 mg BD	Initial dose: 600 mg and 12 hours later, maintenance dose: 400 mg BD	IV: 600 mg every 12 hourly

* optimised dosing dependent upon severity of infection and weight of patient

References

[1] Renal Drug Handbook, 3rd edn. Ashley C and Currie A eds. Radcliffe Publishing Ltd (Oxon), 2009

[2] Electronic Medicines Compendium SPC http://www.medicines.org.uk/emc/ [accessed 11.11.12]

[3] Management of Viral Infection_ Haemopoietic Stem Cell Transplantation Programme (15/06/2010) UCLH Guideline

[4] Pneumocystis Carinii Pneumonia (PCP) Guidelines for the treatment of opportunistic infections in adult HIV positive patients. Camden Provider Services, 2008.

[5] UCLH ICU gentamicin guideline, updated 2009

[6] Bergner R, et al. Fluconazole dosing in continuous veno-venous haemofiltration (CVVHF): need for a high daily dose of 800 mg. *Nephrol Dial Transplant* 2006;21(4):1019–23

[7] Shulman R, et al. UKCPA antiviral management of H1N1 in intensive care, Dec. 2011 version 5

[8] Rybak M, et al. Therapeutic monitoring of vancomycin in adult patients: a consensus review of the American Society of Health-System Pharmacists, the Infectious Diseases Society of America and the Society of Infectious Diseases Pharmacists. *Am J Health Sys Pharm* 2009; 66: 82–98

CHEMICAL PLEURODESIS OF MALIGNANT PLEURAL EFFUSION

Until recently, tetracycline was the most widely used but is now no longer available worldwide. Doxycycline and talc are now the two recommended sclerosing agents. They are thought to work by causing inflammation of the pleural membranes. This procedure can be painful. In the awake patient, administer 15–25 ml lidocaine 1% (maximum dose 3 mg/kg) via the chest drain immediately prior to the sclerosing agent. Intravenous opioids and paracetamol may be required. Anti–inflammatory drugs, such as NSAIDs and steroids, should be avoided for up to 2 days before and after the procedure if possible. Talc has a high success rate and is usually well tolerated. Pleuritic chest pain and mild fever are the commonest side effects. However, ARDS is associated with the use of talc in less than 1% of cases. Doxycycline has no serious complications and tends to be the first choice with talc reserved for recurrent effusions. The major disadvantages of bleomycin are the cost and the need for trained personnel familiar with the handling of cytotoxic drugs.

Procedure
- Ensure drainage of the effusion and lung re–expansion
- Analgesics in the awake patient
- Clamp drain at patient's end and insert 50 ml bladder syringe filled with 3 mg/kg lidocaine (20 ml 1% solution for 70 kg patient)
- Release clamp and inject the lidocaine slowly into the pleural space
- Clamp drain and in the same manner inject either doxycycline 500 mg or talc 2 to 5 g or bleomycin 60000 units (4 vials) diluted in up to 50 ml sodium chloride 0.9% with the bladder syringe
- Flush drain with 10 ml sodium chloride 0.9%
- Clamp the drain for 60 min, observing for signs of increasing pneumothorax (tachycardia, hypotension, falling oxygen saturation, decreased tidal volumes)
- When talc is used, encourage patient to roll onto both sides if possible
- Unclamp the drain and leave on free drainage
- In the absence of excessive fluid drainage (>250 ml/day), the drain should be removed within 3 days of sclerosant administration
- If excessive fluid drainage persists (>250 ml/day), repeat pleurodesis with alternative sclerosant

Sclerosing agent	Dose	Success rate (%)	Side-effects	Cost
Doxycycline	500 mg	76	Chest pain (40%), fever	£23
Talc	2–5 g	90	Chest pain (7%), fever, ARDS (<1%)	4 g £11
Bleomycin	60000 units	61	Chest pain, fever, nausea	£65

Reference: British Thoracic Society Guidelines for the management of malignant pleural effusions. *Thorax* 2003; **58** (suppl II); ii29–ii38.

Appendices

APPENDIX A: CREATININE CLEARANCE

Severity of renal impairment is expressed in terms of glomerular filtration rate, usually measured by creatinine clearance. Creatinine clearance may be estimated from the serum creatinine.

Estimating creatinine clearance from serum creatinine:

For men:

$$CC \ (ml/min) = \frac{weight \ (kg) \times (140 - age) \times 1.23}{serum \ creatinine \ (\mu mol/l)}$$

For women:

$$CC \ (ml/min) = \frac{weight \ (kg) \times (140 - age) \times 1.03}{serum \ creatinine \ (\mu mol/l)}$$

Normal range (based on an adult with a body surface area of 1.73 m^2):

Age	Sex	CC (ml/min)
20–29	Male	94–140
	Female	72–110
30–39	Male	59–137
	Female	71–121

For each decade thereafter values decrease by 6.5 ml/min.

Renal impairment is arbitrarily divided into three grades:

Grade	CC (ml/min)
Mild	20–50
Moderate	10–20
Severe	<10

Renal function declines with age; many elderly patients have a glomerular filtration rate <50 ml/min, which, because of reduced muscle mass, may not be indicated by a raised serum creatinine. It is wise to assume at least mild renal impairment when prescribing for the elderly.

APPENDIX B: WEIGHT CONVERSION (STONES/LB TO KG)

		Lb						
		0	2	4	6	8	10	12	13
S T O N E S	6	38.1	39.0	40.0	40.8	41.7	42.6	43.5	44.0
	7	44.5	45.4	46.3	47.2	48.1	49.0	49.9	50.3
	8	50.8	51.7	52.6	53.5	54.4	55.3	56.2	56.7
	9	57.2	58.1	59.0	59.9	60.8	61.7	62.6	63.0
	10	63.5	64.4	65.3	66.2	67.1	68.0	68.9	69.4
	11	69.9	70.8	71.7	72.6	73.5	74.4	75.4	75.7
	12	76.2	77.1	78.0	78.9	79.8	80.7	81.6	82.1
	13	82.6	83.5	84.4	85.3	86.2	87.0	88.0	88.4
	14	88.9	89.8	90.7	91.6	92.5	93.4	94.3	94.8
	15	95.3	96.2	97.1	98.0	98.9	99.8	100.7	101.1
	16	101.6	102.5	103.4	104.3	105.2	106.1	107.0	107.5
	17	108.0	108.9	109.8	110.7	111.6	112.5	113.4	113.8
	18	114.3	115.2	116.1	117.0	117.9	118.8	119.7	120.2

APPENDIX C: BODY MASS INDEX (BMI) CALCULATOR

$$BMI = \frac{Weight\ (kg)}{Height\ (m)^2}$$

To use the table:

First convert weight to kg (1 lb = 0.45 kg).

Then read across from patient's height until you reach the weight (kg) nearest to the patient's.

Then read up the chart to obtain the BMI.

Height											
Feet/ inches	Metres	20	21	22	23	24	25	26	27	28	29	30
5'0"	1.52	46	49	51	53	55	58	60	62	65	67	69
5'1"	1.55	48	50	53	55	58	60	62	65	67	70	72
5'2"	1.58	50	52	55	57	60	62	65	67	70	72	75
5'3"	1.60	51	54	56	59	61	64	67	69	72	74	77
5'4"	1.63	53	56	58	61	64	66	69	72	74	77	80
5'5"	1.65	54	57	60	63	65	68	71	74	76	79	82
5'6"	1.68	56	59	62	65	68	71	73	76	79	82	85
5'7"	1.70	58	61	64	66	69	72	75	78	81	84	87
5'8"	1.73	60	63	66	69	72	75	78	81	84	87	90
5'9"	1.75	61	64	67	70	74	77	80	83	86	89	92
5'10"	1.78	63	67	70	73	76	79	82	86	89	92	95
5'11"	1.80	65	68	71	75	78	81	84	87	91	94	97
6'0"	1.83	67	70	74	77	80	84	87	90	94	97	100
6'1"	1.85	68	72	75	79	82	86	89	92	96	99	103
6'2"	1.88	71	74	78	81	85	88	92	95	99	102	106
6'3"	1.90	72	76	79	83	87	90	94	97	101	105	108
6'4"	1.93	74	78	82	86	89	93	97	101	104	108	112
6'5"	1.96	77	80	84	88	92	96	99	103	107	111	115
		Desirable						Moderately obese				

<20 = underweight

20–24.9 = desirable

25–29.9 = moderately obese

>30 = obese

APPENDIX D: LEAN BODY WEIGHT CHARTS

For men:

Height in feet & inches (cm)	Weight (kg)		
	Small frame	Medium frame	Large frame
5'6" (168)	62–65	63–69	66–75
5'7" (170)	63–66	65–70	68–76
5'8" (173)	64–67	66–71	69–78
5'9" (175)	65–68	69–74	70–80
5'10" (178)	65–70	69–74	72–82
5'11" (180)	66–71	70–75	73–84
6'0" (183)	68–73	71–77	75–85
6'1" (185)	69–75	73–79	76–87
6'2" (188)	70–76	75–81	78–90
6'3" (191)	72–78	76–83	80–92
6'4" (193)	74–80	78–85	82–94

For women:

Height in feet & inches (cm)	Weight (kg)		
	Small frame	Medium frame	Large frame
5'0" (152)	47–52	51–57	55–62
5'1" (155)	48–54	52–59	57–64
5'2" (158)	49–55	54–60	58–65
5'3" (160)	50–56	55–61	60–67
5'4" (163)	52–58	56–63	61–69
5'5" (165)	53–59	58–64	62–70
5'6" (168)	55–60	59–65	64–72
5'7" (170)	56–62	60–67	65–74
5'8" (173)	57–63	62–68	66–76
5'9" (175)	59–65	63–70	68–77
5'10" (178)	60–66	65–71	69–79
5'11" (180)	61–67	66–72	70–80
6'0" (183)	63–69	67–74	72–81

APPENDIX E: INFUSION RATE/ DOSE CALCULATION

To calculate the infusion rate in ml/h:

$$\text{Infusion rate (ml/h)} = \frac{\text{Dose } (\mu g/kg/min) \times \text{Weight (kg)} \times 60}{\text{Concentration of solution } (\mu g/ml)}$$

To calculate the dose in $\mu g/kg/min$:

$$\text{Dose } (\mu g/kg/min) = \frac{\text{Infusion rate (ml/h)} \times \text{Concentration of solution } (\mu g/ml)}{\text{Weight (kg)} \times 60}$$

For example: adrenaline infusion (4 mg made up to 50 ml) running at 6 ml/h in a patient weighing 80 kg:

$$\text{Dose } (\mu g/kg/min) = \frac{6 \text{ ml/h} \times \dfrac{4000 \ \mu g}{50 \text{ ml}}}{80 \text{ (kg)} \times 60}$$

$$= 0.1 \ \mu g/kg/min$$

APPENDIX F: DRUG COMPATIBILITY CHART

Ideally, all drugs given intravenously should be given via a dedicated line or lumen, and not mixed at any stage. However, if this is not possible, then compatibility data must be obtained before co-administering drugs. In general, drugs should not be added to parenteral nutrition, or to blood products. Sodium bicarbonate and mannitol solutions should not be used as diluent for intravenous drug administration.

As a general guide, line compatibility of different drugs often depends on the pH of the drugs concerned. This will vary depending on how the drug is reconstituted or diluted. Drugs with widely differing pH will almost certainly be incompatible. However, the converse is not necessarily true, and lines should always be checked regularly for any gross signs of incompatibility (e.g. precipitate formation).

This chart indicates whether two drugs can be run in through the same IV access. It assumes normal concentrations and infusion rates for each drug, and data may vary depending on the diluent used. It should be used as a guide only, and not taken as definitive.

Please refer to the folded table at the back of the book.

APPENDIX G: OMEPRAZOLE ADMINISTRATION RECORD

York Hospitals **NHS**

NHS Trust

Prescription chart for omeprazole infusion

This regimen gives an omeprazole dose of 80 mg iv over 1 hour (given as 2 x 40 mg each over 30 minutes), then a continuous infusion of 8 mg/h for 72 hours.

Notes.

• Ensure you have the correct omeprazole preparation i.e. infusion NOT injection

• Omeprazole vial is compatible with a 100 ml minibag plus of sodium chloride 0.9%

ENTER KNOWN DRUG ALLERGIES/ SENSITIVITIES OR WRITE NIL KNOWN	First Name:	
	Surname:	
	D.O.B.:	
Dr's Signature:	Bleep:	Hosp. No:
N.B. PATIENT MUST HAVE RED ALLERGY BAND IN SITU	Consultant	Weight

Date	Route	Infusion fluid	Volume	Additions to Infusion		Time to run or ml/hour	Prescriber's signature	Batch no.	Actual start time & date	Signature		Asset no. of pump: (if used)
				Drug	**Dose**					Administered by	Checked by	
	IV	Sodium chloride 0.9%	100 ml	Omeprazole	40 mg	30 min (200 ml/h)						
	IV	Sodium chloride 0.9%	100 ml	Omeprazole	40 mg	30 min (200 ml/h)						
	IV	Sodium chloride 0.9%	100 ml	Omeprazole	40 mg	5 h (20 ml/h)						

(Continued)

								5 h (20 ml/h)	40 mg	Omeprazole	100 ml	Sodium chloride 0.9%	IV
								5 h (20 ml/h)	40 mg	Omeprazole	100 ml	Sodium chloride 0.9%	IV
								5 h (20 ml/h)	40 mg	Omeprazole	100 ml	Sodium chloride 0.9%	IV
								5 h (20 ml/h)	40 mg	Omeprazole	100 ml	Sodium chloride 0.9%	IV
								5 h (20 ml/h)	40 mg	Omeprazole	100 ml	Sodium chloride 0.9%	IV
								5 h (20 ml/h)	40 mg	Omeprazole	100 ml	Sodium chloride 0.9%	IV
								5 h (20 ml/h)	40 mg	Omeprazole	100 ml	Sodium chloride 0.9%	IV
								5 h (20 ml/h)	40 mg	Omeprazole	100 ml	Sodium chloride 0.9%	IV
								5 h (20 ml/h)	40 mg	Omeprazole	100 ml	Sodium chloride 0.9%	IV
								5 h (20 ml/h)	40 mg	Omeprazole	100 ml	Sodium chloride 0.9%	IV
								5 h (20 ml/h)	40 mg	Omeprazole	100 ml	Sodium chloride 0.9%	IV
								5 h (20 ml/h)	40 mg	Omeprazole	100 ml	Sodium chloride 0.9%	IV
								5 h (20 ml/h)	40 mg	Omeprazole	100 ml	Sodium chloride 0.9%	IV
								5 h (20 ml/h)	40 mg	Omeprazole	100 ml	Sodium chloride 0.9%	IV

APPENDIX H: SODIUM CONTENT OF ORAL MEDICATIONS

The normal daily requirement of sodium for an adult is 100 mmol. ICU patients are frequently administered effervescent or soluble tablets and these can contribute a significant sodium load. Below is a list of commonly used oral medications in the ICU with their sodium content. The precise values given for generic products may differ slightly between manufacturers.

Preparation	Approximate sodium content, per dose unit
Aciclovir 200 mg/400 mg/800 mg tabs (manufacturer Actavis)	<1 mmol
Aspirin 75 mg dispersible tabs	<1 mmol
Co-beneldopa (Madopar®) 62.5 mg/ 125 mg dispersible tablets	None
Co-codamol 8/500 dispersible/ effervescent/soluble tablets	16.7–19 mmol per tablet
Diclofenac (Voltarol®) 50 mg dispersible tablets	<1 mmol
Gastrocote® liquid	2.1 mmol in 5 ml
Lansoprazole (Zoton® FasTab®) orodispersible tablets	None
Mirtazipine 15 mg/30 mg/45 mg orodispersible tablets	None
Olanzapine 5 mg/10 mg/15 mg/20 mg orodispersible tablets	None
Paracetamol 500 mg soluble tablets	16.9–19.1 mmol per tablet
Phosphate-Sandoz® effervescent tablets	20.4 mmol per tablet
Piroxicam (Feldene Melt®) 20 mg orodispersible tablets	None
Potassium effervescent tablets (Sando-K)	0.1 mmol per tablet
Prednisolone soluble tablets	1.5 mmol per tablet
Ranitidine 150 mg effervescent tablets	5.2 mmol per tablet
Risperidone 0.5 mg/1 mg/2 mg/3 mg/ 4 mg generic orodispersible tablets	None
Sandocal-400® effervescent tablets	None

(Continued)

Sandocal-1000® effervescent tablets	6 mmol per tablet
Sodium bicarbonate 500 mg capsules	6 mmol per capsule
Tramadol (Zamadol Melt®) 50 mg orodispersible tablets	None
Zinc (Solvazinc®) effervescent tablets	4.6 mmol per tablet

Source: National Electronic Library for Medicines

APPENDIX I: DRUG MANAGEMENT OF THE BRAIN-STEM-DEAD DONOR

- Initially, **methylprednisolone** 15 mg/kg IV bolus, as soon as possible. Methylprednisolone is associated with reduced lung water and renders the lungs more suitable for transplant
- Continue **antibiotics** as indicated
- **Insulin** ≥1 unit/hour, blood glucose target 4–9 mmol/l
- **Inotropes and vasopressors** may be indicated (p. 277). If response to catecholamine infusion is inadequate, a trial of **hydrocortisone** 50–100 mg intravenously may improve cardiovascular parameters
- Diabetes insipidus is a common problem and may need treatment with **vasopressin** (p. 234) or **desmopressin (DDAVP)** (p. 70)
- Recent studies suggest that **tri-iodothyronine** (T_3) supplementation may add little to an intensive donor management protocol which includes vasopressin and methylprednisolone, and suggest using it only if cardiac performance is unresponsive to volume loading and vasopressors. **Tri-iodothyronine** (T_3) 4 µg IV bolus, followed by IV infusion of 3 µg/h
- If hypernatraemia is a problem, use Ringer's lactate solution (**Hartmann's**) or a **glucose-containing** solution. Glucose solution and methylprednisolone may lead to hyperglycaemia, requiring an increase in insulin infusion
- Electrolyte disturbance with low **potassium**, **magnesium**, **calcium** or **phosphate** should be corrected
- Bradycardia will be unresponsive to atropine, use **isoprenaline** or **dobutamine** infusion
- Maintenance **intravenous fluids** should be limited if ongoing losses are not excessive; enteral route can be considered

APPENDIX J: VANCOMYCIN BY CONTINUOUS INFUSION

Underdosing and problems associated with the sampling and the timing of serum level monitoring are problems which may result in decreased efficacy of vancomycin in the treatment of infection. The efficacy of vancomycin depends on the time for which the serum level exceeds the MIC (minimum inhibitory concentration) for the micro-organism rather than on the attainment of high peak levels. Administration of vancomycin as a continuous infusion is therefore an ideal method of administration for optimum efficacy. Once the infusion reaches a steady state, the timing for serum level monitoring is not crucial, and samples can be taken at any time.

Administration – day one

Weight-related loading dose followed immediately by continuous infusion.

IV loading dose:

<70 kg: OR   1 g in 100 ml sodium chloride 0.9% over 2 h via central line

1 g in 250 ml sodium chloride 0.9% over 2 h via peripheral line

≥70 kg: 1.25 g 100 ml sodium chloride 0.9% over 2 h via central OR 1.25 g in 250 ml sodium chloride 0.9% over 2 h via peripheral line

IV infusion:

The continuous intravenous infusion (over 24 h) should follow immediately after the loading dose. The starting dose is based on an estimate of the patient's renal function (see table below).

For central administration: reconstitute 500 mg vancomycin in 10 ml WFI, and further dilute with sodium chloride 0.9% to make up to 50 ml total volume.

For peripheral administration: reconstitute 500 mg vancomycin in 10 ml WFI, and further dilute with sodium chloride 0.9% to make up to 100 ml total volume.

Renal function	Starting vancomycin infusion dose (g; over 24 hours)
Normal (serum creatinine <120 µmol/l)	1.5
Impaired (serum creatinine >120 µmol/l)	1
CVVH	1

Measure serum levels every day at 06:00 hours from day 2 onwards, and adjust dose according to levels (see overleaf).

Adjustment of daily infusion dose – day 2 onwards.

The adjustment of the infusion dose is dependent on the vancomycin level (see following table).

Vancomycin level (mg/l)	Dosage change required	Rate adjustment
<15	Increase the dose by 500 mg	Increase infusion rate to next level up in subsequent table
15–25	No change	No change
>25	Decrease the dose by 500 mg*	Reduce infusion rate to next level down in subsequent table
>30	Stop infusion for minimum of 6 h	Restart at a reduced dose

* If the patient is receiving only 500 mg/day, the dose should be decreased to 250 mg/day (as outlined in table below)

	Infusion rate (ml/h)	
Vancomycin daily dose	via central line (500 mg in 50 ml)	via peripheral line (500 mg in 100 ml)
2.5 g	10.4	20.8
2 g	8.3	16.7
1.5 g	6.3	12.5
1 g	4.2	8.3
500 mg	2.1	4.2
250 mg	1.1	2.1

APPENDIX K: CHILD–PUGH SCORE

The Child–Pugh score is used to assess the prognosis of chronic liver disease, mainly cirrhosis. Although it was originally used to predict mortality during surgery, it is now used to determine the prognosis, as well as the required strength of treatment and the necessity of liver transplantation. This score is to guide dose reduction in liver failure for certain drugs, such as caspofungin and tigecycline.

Scoring

The score employs five clinical measures of liver disease. Each measure is scored 1–3, with 3 indicating most severe derangement.

Measure	1 point	2 points	3 points
Bilirubin (μmol/l)	<34	34–50	>50
Serum albumin (g/l)	>35	28–35	<28
INR	<1.7	1.71–2.20	>2.20
Ascites	None	Suppressed with medication	Refractory
Hepatic encephalopathy	None	Grade I–II (or suppressed	Grade III–IV (or refractory)

In primary sclerosing cholangitis (PSC) and primary biliary cirrhosis (PBC), the bilirubin references are changed to reflect the fact that these diseases feature high conjugated bilirubin levels. The upper limit for 1 point is 68 μmol/l and the upper limit for 2 points is 170 μmol/l.

Interpretation

Chronic liver disease is classified into Child–Pugh classes A to C, employing the added score from above.

Points	Class	One-year survival (%)	Two-year survival (%)
5–6	A	100	85
7–9	B	81	57
10–15	C	45	35

APPENDIX L: SEVERE SEPSIS ALGORITHM

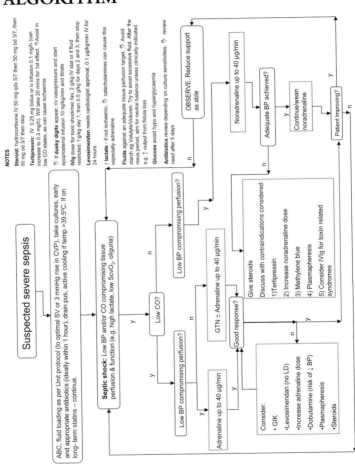

NOTES

Steroid: hydrocortisone IV 50 mg qds 5/7 then 50 mg bd 3/7, then 50 mg od 3/7 then stop

Terlipressin: IV 0.25 mg bolus or iv infusion 0.1 mg/h (can increase to 0.3 mg/h). Will take 20 mins for 1st effect. ⟳ Avoid in low CO states, as can cause ischaemia

⟳ If **dusky digits** appear, n/v vasopressors and start epoprostenol infusion 10 ng/kg/min and titrate

IVIg dose for toxic shock/nec fas: 2 g/kg IV stat or if fluid restricted: 1 g/kg day 1, then 0.5 g/kg for days 2 and 3, then stop

Levosimendan needs cardiologist approval. 0.1 µg/kg/min IV for 24 hours

↑ **lactate** - if not ischaemic, ⟳ catecholamines can cause this especially adrenaline

Fluids against an adequate tissue perfusion target. ⟳ Avoid starch eg Volulyte/Voluven. Try to avoid excessive fluid. After the resus period, aim for neutral balance unless clinically indicated e.g. ↑ output from fistula loss

Glucose avoid hypo and hyperglycaemia

Antibiotics review depending on culture sensitivities. ⟳ review need after 5 days

Suspected severe sepsis

ABC, fluid loading as per Unit protocol (to optimal SV or 3 mmHg rise in CVP), take cultures, early and appropriate antibiotics (ideally within 1 hour), drain pus, active cooling if temp >39.5°C. If on long-term statins – continue.

Septic shock: Low BP and/or CO compromising tissue perfusion & function (e.g. high lactate, low ScvO₂, oliguria)

Low CO?

Low BP compromising perfusion?

Low BP compromising perfusion?

Adrenaline up to 40 µg/min

GTN ± Adrenaline up to 40 µg/min

Low BP compromising perfusion?

Good response?

Consider:
• GIK
• Levosimendan (no LD)
• Increase adrenaline dose
• Dobutamine (risk of ↓ BP)
• Plasmapheresis
• Steroids

Give steroids

Discuss with contraindications considered:
1) Terlipressin
2) Increase noradrenaline dose
3) Methylene blue
4) Plasmapheresis
5) Consider IVIg for toxin related syndromes

Noradrenaline up to 40 µg/min

Adequate BP achieved?

Continue/wean noradrenaline

OBSERVE. Reduce support as able

Patient improving?

DRUG INDEX

Proprietary (trade) names are printed in *italics*.

DRUG INDEX